A Taste of Heaven and Earth

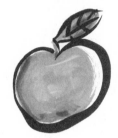

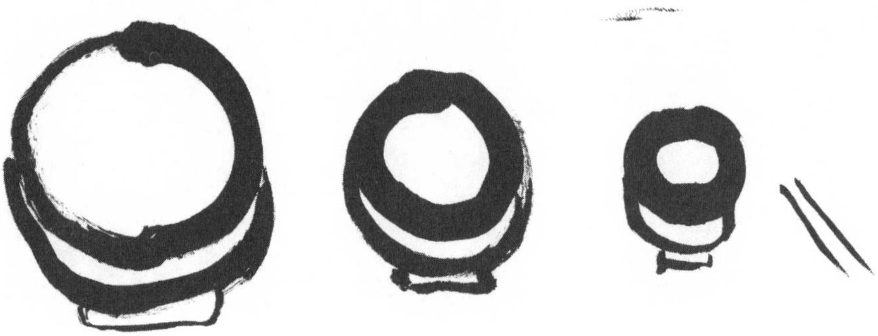

A Taste of Heaven and Earth

Bettina Vitell

Illustrations by Susan Morningstar

HarperPerennial
A Division of HarperCollins *Publishers*

HarperCollins books may be purchased for educational, business, or sales promotional use. For information, please write: Special Markets Department, HarperCollins Publishers, Inc., 10 East 53rd Street, New York, NY 10022.

"Sensory Awareness: The Rediscovery of Experiencing" is reprinted with permission from the author, Kenneth McCarthy, and was published in the *Yoga Journal*, September 1987.

FIRST EDITION

Designed by David Bullen
Composition by Wilsted & Taylor

Library of Congress Cataloging-in-Publication Data

Vitell, Bettina.
    A taste of heaven and earth: a Zen approach to cooking and eating with 150 satisfying vegetarian recipes / Bettina Vitell; illustrations by Susan Morningstar.
       p.   cm.
    Includes index.
    ISBN 0-06-055333-2 — ISBN 0-06-096934-2 (pbk.)
     1. Vegetarian cookery.   2. Cookery—Religious aspects—Zen Buddhism.   I. Title.
TX837.V58   1993
641.5'636—dc20   92-56253

93 94 95 96 97 RRD 10 9 8 7 6 5 4 3 2 1

95 96 97 RRD 10 9 8 7 6 5   (pbk.)

With deep gratitude this book is dedicated
to my teachers
Eido Shimano Roshi and Charlotte Selver

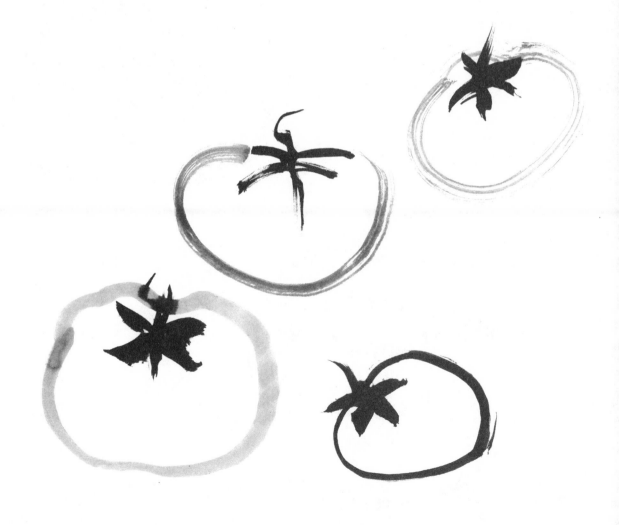

UMMONS CARE

JOSHU'S TEA

Contents

Soups

Pasta and Grains

Curries

Mexican Tastes

Sushi Ideas

Pizzas and Vegetable Tarts

Vegetable Dishes

Salads

Sauces and Salad Dressings

Breakfast Ideas

Desserts

Acknowledgments

This book would never have been written without Kenneth McCarthy. In many ways it is his book, although he has never cooked a thing in his life; he's a great writer and worked with me from beginning to end on the words and phrasing of this book. Practically every recipe has been tested on his culinary and discriminating tastes as well. Julia Child, in her book *Mastering the Art of French Cooking*, applauds her friends for being "guinea pigs" for her recipes, and I applaud Ken for putting up with endless meals, some delicious, some not, and what seemed like endless work clarifying most of what is written here.

My family read the first drafts and encouraged me every step of the way. I thank my mother and father especially for their creative minds and passionate natures; my sister Zizi and my aunt and uncle, Joan and Rod Perkins, for their boundless enthusiasm and support.

John Vitell and The Beat'n Path Cafe taught me about dedication and commitment. Thanks to the many cooks, waitresses, waiters, bartenders, and customers of the Beat'n Path who in their own way contributed to this book.

Susan Morningstar, one of the best cooks I know, has shared many of her ideas, complete with a quirky sense of humor. Having long admired her zenga-style painting, I am very grateful for her illustrations in this book.

Many thanks to my dearest cooking partners at Dai Bosatsu; to Jiun Ewa Tarasewicz and Hisen Tracy LaRock for teaching me much about the heart of cooking; and to Ho-on Chris Adamo for always being steadfast and calm in the kitchen.

I am grateful to all the participants in the 1990 Sensory Awareness Leader's Group, who cooked with me at our study retreat and directly inspired this book: Jill Harris, Lilith Pincus, Ron Riley, Athanasia Chronis, Martina Hornstien, Louise Boedeker, Krista Sattler, Julie Esterly-Morgan, Monika Zitta, Pat Meyer, Ray Fowler, Mary Connelly, Margrit Strauli, Penny Smith, Helga Hoenen, Seymour Carter, Terry Ray, and Gordon Bennett.

I am particularly thankful to Michael Katz, my agent, for seeing the possibilities in this book and helping to make them a reality. I am very grateful to my editor, Susan Friedland, who took a manuscript that was unruly and with great skill shaped it into a book.

A Taste of Heaven and Earth is also dedicated to the memory of my friend Donge John Haber. He was a passionate cook, a wonderful gardener, a director of opera, and a Zen monk who dedicated his life to others.

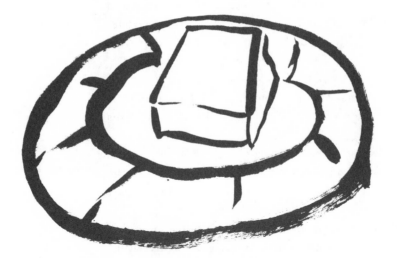

TOFU ON ZAFU

Foreword

I would like to introduce both the author and the artist of this book. The author, Chika Bettina Vitell, has been my student for more than ten years in both New York Zendo in Manhattan and Dai Bosatsu Zendo in the Catskills. She has a profound interest in Japanese culture and therefore such historical names as Dogen, Hakuin, Basho, and Rikyu appear. At one time I thought she had been born in America by mistake, but now I think that she was meant to be born here. She has combined her interests in American and Japanese culture, Zen, Tea, and Haiku and has long practiced cooking for western students with a bicultural taste. This book is a manifestation of those interests.

She is quite an elusive individual in one sense; in another sense, she is vividly everywhere. So she concentrated her intense energy on *A Taste of Heaven and Earth*. As much as the kitchen is a place of transformation, the zendo is a place of spiritual transformation. As a result of her years of Zen practice and Tea, she has learned to think from her belly and her intuition has been sharpened. This, after all, is what this book is all about.

The artist of this book, Seiko Susan Morningstar, is also my student and was ordained last year as a Rinzai Buddhist nun. Right now she is practicing at Dai Bosatsu Zendo. In Seiko's case, her artwork is her "cooking." I find it so appropriate that she has done the illustrations for this cookbook, since one of her other gifts is for growing things in the earth. For more than two years she was the resident student at New York Zendo where, amid many other duties, she applied her artist's eye to the care of our garden. She continues her artistic and gardening practices at the monastery.

No masterpiece feast can be measured by two spoons of this, one sugar of that; it's all done by intuition. It is the intuitive reflection between artist and author that makes this book so special. Their beautiful dharma friendship has been a mirror; the fusion of their talents is this book.

I am so pleased with the publication of *A Taste of Heaven and Earth*, as we have been waiting at least twenty years to have this kind of guide. It is an excellent introduction to simple, delicious, healthy, and beautiful vegetarian food. As the world gets more and more complicated, more and more polluted, what we now need most is simplicity and a natural lifestyle.

I am convinced that if we combine the careful preparation of food with about an hour of Zen meditation practice every day, we will have a peaceful and contented life. What more, after all, do we need?

Eido Tai Shimano Roshi
Abbot, Dai Bosatsu Zendo
April 1992

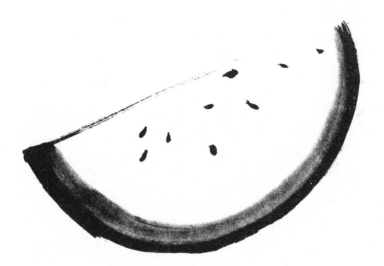

EAT THE
MELON
WITHOUT
OPENING
YOUR MOUTH

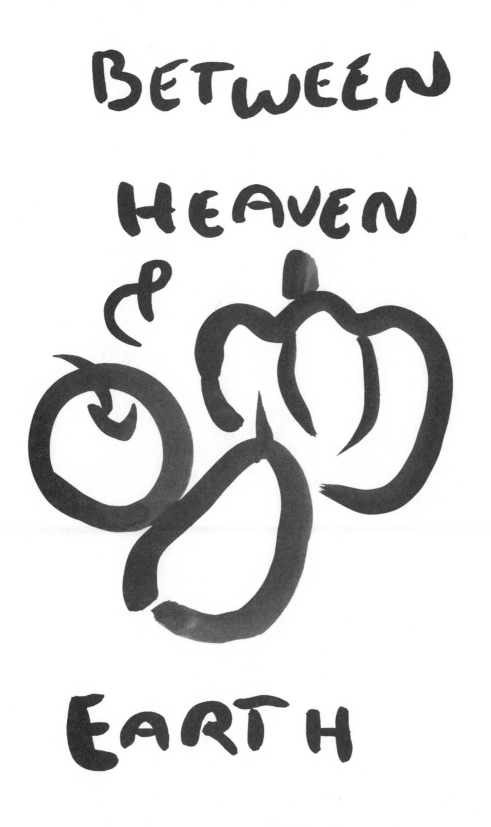

BETWEEN

HEAVEN

&

EARTH

Introduction

The kitchen is a place of transformation: a place where tomatoes, fresh from the garden, become a sauce for pasta; where black beans combined with fiery spices become chili, and flour mixed with yeast and honey becomes bread. As cooks, we bring together fresh vegetables, spices from around the world, whole grains and beans, fruits and nuts, and transform them into heartwarming meals.

This book is about another kind of transformation as well. Like many cookbooks, it is filled with delicious recipes, but unlike any cookbook that I know of, it talks about the cook too.

We cook with spices to make our food lively. We use tender lettuces to make salads that refresh us. When it's cold outside, we cook warm, hearty stews to give us strength. But food is not the only thing that nurtures us. The way we prepare our food and the wholeheartedness we bring to each moment of cooking nurtures us too.

Human beings are creatures of action, and it's through action that we reveal ourselves and come to know our deepest nature. What creates happiness and vitality? How can we become more peaceful? What ingredients do we need for a rich and full life? We can explore these and other questions just as a cook creates a new recipe—by experimenting with subtle flavors and essences.

Zen practice is at the core of my cooking. After years of owning my own restaurant, The Beat'n Path Cafe, I spent a year as Tenzo, or head cook, at Dai Bosatsu Zendo, a traditional Rinzai Zen monastery in the Catskill Mountains of New York. I'd been a Zen student for many years in New York, and cooking was a natural outgrowth of my meditation practice. In the Zen tradition, serving as Tenzo is considered an excellent opportunity for practice. The literature of Zen is filled with kitchen anecdotes and stories of enlightenment coming through simple daily chores.

Dai Bosatsu Zendo is an authentic Japanese-style Zen temple set at the end of a long dirt road, deep in the Catskills next to a large serene lake. There's also a rambling old Victorian house on the property where guests stay during the summer for retreats and workshops.

Many of the recipes in this book were cooked for the guests and students. Some came to meditate; others, to enjoy the quiet atmosphere and natural beauty. I have wonderful memories of early mornings in the kitchen with the smell of fresh baked apricot muffins and hot coffee filling the air. The mist is rising from the lake and I hear the temple bell echoing across the mountains.

But not all my cooking has been in such a rarefied environment.

My first real job as a cook was on the tugboat *Philip T. Feeney*, which towed barges up the Erie Canal from New York City to Niagara Falls. The galley was tiny and had just two small refrigerators, three by three feet each. To give you an idea of the life-style on board the boat, one of the refrigerators held nothing but six-packs of beer! Nutritious food was not a priority. Nevertheless, I managed to cook splendid vegetarian meals, which the crew loved. But whenever we docked at a town along the way, they wasted no time going "up the street" for a good hamburger.

After the glories of cruising the Erie Canal, I found myself working as a sauté and broiler cook at one of New York City's first vegetarian restaurants. John Lennon and Yoko Ono used to come in almost every day for lunch and I would cook special meals for them. The East West Restaurant was an exciting place to be, but it was hard, hard work. Along with my stylish chef's uniform and my huge white chef's hat, I wore heavy work boots. Within six months, the tough leather boots were completely worn out.

The pace was dizzying. It wasn't unusual for me to have six sauté pans going on the stove at once. I quickly became expert at flipping pans of scallops, shrimp, and vegetables in the air, followed by great licks of flame.

It was there, at East West, that I began to appreciate the power of my senses. Given the speed with which we had to work, there was a tangible element of danger in the kitchen. With huge pans of boiling water, hot oil, and fire everywhere, it was no place to daydream. I learned to hear not only with my ears and feel not only with my hands but with my whole self.

The cooking experience that inspired this book took place in the summer of 1990. My friend and teacher Charlotte Selver invited me to cook for a six-week workshop she was giving at a retreat center in northern California. Charlotte is one of the pioneers of the Human Potential Movement. Her practice, Sensory Awareness, which she has been offering for more than fifty years, has had a deep influence on people like Erich Fromm, Fritz Perls, and Alan Watts.

Sensory Awareness is a practice that deepens and clarifies all our experiences. What better place to study than in a lively kitchen? Smelling the aroma of a simmering soup, feeling the coolness of water when washing lettuce, tasting a fresh basil leaf—all these things became an extension of our classes.

The students took turns cooking together, and we used many of the recipes that are now in this book. We would often come directly into the kitchen from classes to begin lunch or dinner. The food we cooked was wonderful, and our experience of working together was so inspiring that it seems only fitting to include in this book some of the elements of our study.

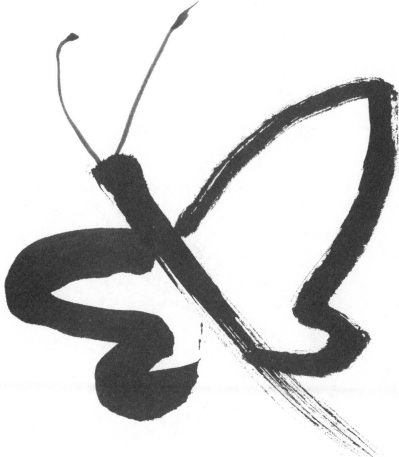

This cookbook is filled with recipes for delicious meals, but it's also a book that asks questions. I offer these questions to you as a way both to taste some of what I have discovered in the kitchen and to encourage you to make your own discoveries. What is the source of your aliveness? What brings you greater clarity? What leads you to a more connected and aware way of living?

There is more to cooking than meets the eye.

Dogen Zenji, a famous Zen master of the thirteenth century, considered the practice of cooking to be so important that he wrote these profound instructions for his cooks to follow. They speak directly to us:

When you prepare food, do not see with ordinary eyes and do not think with ordinary mind. Take up a blade of grass and construct a treasure king's land; enter into a particle of dust and turn the great dharma wheel. Do not arouse disdainful mind when you prepare a broth of wild grasses; do not arouse joyful mind when you prepare a fine cream soup.

This is the way to turn things while being turned by things. Keep yourself harmonious and wholehearted in this way and do not lose one eye, or two eyes.

Take up a green vegetable and turn it into a sixteen-foot golden body; take up a sixteen-foot golden body and turn it into a green vegetable leaf.

This is a miraculous transformation—a work that benefits sentient beings.

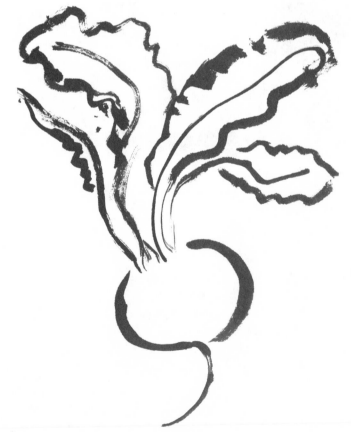

Kitchen Notes

The recipes in this book are influenced by the foods of Mexico, Thailand, Japan, Italy, India, and the southwestern United States. Many of the ingredients come from around the world: tofu, soy sauce, curry spices, coconut milk, salsas, and tortillas. They can be found easily in large supermarkets.

Inspiration comes from the splendid variety of fresh fruits and vegetables being grown on small farms around the country. Our markets carry purple potatoes and yellow beets, white eggplants and orange bell peppers, and chilis in all shapes and sizes. Chicories and radicchio are commonplace, and such fresh herbs as cilantro and basil can be found year round.

The cooking in this book reflects an understanding of the relationship between food and health. The American diet is changing rapidly: away from meat and dairy products. As we become more educated about our health, we find that food can be healing. When we need more vitamin A, we can eat fresh mustard greens and broccoli. Whole grains are good for the immune system, and beans provide us with a low cholesterol protein. The notes that follow (and the menus in the appendix on page 207) will give you some kitchen tips for creating healthy and delicious food as well as some ideas for planning your menus.

First and foremost: Taste your cooking. Recipes are just the bare bones. Good cooking comes from asking questions and being curious. Trust yourself. Be inventive and take chances.

Become familiar with the tastes of your ingredients, especially seasonings. Many of the directions in the recipes call for seasoning *to taste*. This is the fun of cooking: making your choices and savoring the flavors you create. Add lemon and lime juice, ginger, chili peppers, salt, tamari, fresh herbs, and spices carefully as you go along, a little at a time; too much seasoning is difficult to remedy.

If you like black bean chili hot and spicy, add more jalapeños than the recipe calls for. If you love the taste of ginger, add more of it to your dishes. The recipes in this book are designed so you can follow your tastes to create meals that are fun and rewarding to cook.

Plan your menus ahead, but be flexible according to the mood of the day, the weather, and the season. Cook according to what is happening around you and the people you are cooking for. In the winter serve stews, thick soups, casseroles, and hot cereals in the mornings. If your friends are engaged in strenuous work and it's cold outside, make them something hardy and warm spirited like a spicy chili or a curry stew.

In the summer you naturally want to eat lightly. Serve more fruits and salads. Gardens are filled with lettuces, herbs, and an abundance of young, tender vegetables. Use ingredients that are fresh, and your meals will always have a vibrant quality to them.

Presentation is important. Vegetarian cooking is colorful. Red beets are brilliant in a salad of dark, luminous green spinach. A sauce of tomatoes, red peppers, carrots, and acorn squash is lovely with yellow polenta. Fruits mixed together in salads sparkle like jewels.

Garnishes add the finishing touch to your dish. Simple garnishes such as chopped parsley, chopped nuts, or minced red peppers can be sprinkled on top of a dish. Or place a small mound of thinly sliced purple cabbage or a tiny bouquet of watercress on the side of each plate. Edible flowers look beautiful scattered in a salad. Here is another opportunity to experiment, using your sense of design, pattern, and color to make beautiful food.

Vegetarian cooks are constantly chopping and slicing all sorts of ingredients. Keep your knives sharp and learn how to be skillful with them. It's a great art. When I was in the restaurant business and had to interview new cooks for a chef's position, I would give them an enormous onion and ask them to slice it. In an instant, I would know how experienced they were.

Good preparation is important. Keep your work area clean and neat. This will keep your mind clear and make your job easier. Have you ever had the experience of trying to find your way in a cluttered kitchen? It's confusing, and it seems like you are always one step behind, trying to catch up.

Get in the habit of cleaning up as you go along. When you finish one task, wipe your cutting board clean. Put everything away that you no longer need. Then start again with space and clarity around you. The care that you bring to your preparation is an important ingredient in cooking, and can be savored in the meals you make.

Leftovers are an invitation to be creative. Generally the best ideas come when you open the refrigerator, take a look at what's available, and use your cooking instincts to invent something new. Many of the recipes in this book were created in just this way.

Extra vegetables can always be stir-fried with rice. Leftover baked potatoes can be made into potato salad. Extra curried vegetables can be mixed with rice for a pilaf salad. The cooking broth from beans makes a wonderful stock for soups.

The colors and tastes of your ingredients will inspire you. And even if what you make is not the perfect dish, you will still learn from it.

Cooking mindfully means seeing beyond the kitchen and realizing that whatever you do affects the whole.

There are many ways to contribute to the world. As cooks, you can recycle your bottles and cans, buy goods packaged in recycled paper, and bring home groceries in cloth bags.

And whenever you buy organic food, you cast your vote for an agriculture that supports your health, the health of the people who grow your food, and the health of the earth. It's a vote for life.

Many markets are now carrying organic produce. It's not much more expensive and it tastes much better. There is an organic market in my neighborhood filled with the most beautiful array of produce I have ever seen. As I pass by, I can't resist stopping in just to look at the new vegetables and fruits that appear each day. It's like visiting an art gallery. Someday these markets will be commonplace.

Cooking Techniques

How to Use Ginger: Choose fresh gingerroot that is firm and not wrinkled. Use a small paring knife to peel away the skin, then grate finely. If you are using a lot of ginger, peel it, cut it into small pieces, and grate it in an electric nut grinder.

Ginger juice is used often in the recipes. Finely grate the ginger, then wrap it in a thin towel and squeeze the juice through the cloth into a small cup. Discard the ginger pulp.

How to Cook Beans: Many people think beans are hard to digest and cause gas. There is a simple cooking remedy for this. First, sort through the beans to remove stones. An easy and fast way to do this is to pour ¼ cup of beans at a time onto a white saucer. You will spot stones immediately. Discard them.

Rinse the beans thoroughly, then place them in a pot with enough fresh water to just cover them. Bring to a rolling boil. Remove from the heat, drain the water, and rinse the beans again. Place the thoroughly rinsed beans in a pot of fresh water. The ratio of beans to water is 1 : 3. Bring again to a boil. Cover with a lid, reduce the heat, and simmer the beans until they are soft.

How to Cook Rice: A heavy pot is the key to making perfect, fluffy rice. It should distribute the heat evenly and have a tight-fitting lid. The proportion of rice to water is 1 : 2, 1 cup of rice to 2 cups of water.

Always rinse the rice in cold water before cooking. Add the rice and water to the pot, cover with a tight lid, and bring to a boil. When steam escapes from the lid, immediately turn the heat to low and simmer for 40 minutes.

How to Use Dry Mushrooms: When cooking with dry shiitake or dry porcini mushrooms, the procedure is the same. Cover the mushrooms amply with water and soak for at least half an hour before cooking, until they become soft. Drain, then squeeze them dry with your hands. Remove the stems and prepare the mushrooms as per instructions in the recipe. The stems can be used for making soup stock. Wrap them in a plastic bag and refrigerate for up to a week.

How to Prepare Tofu: Tofu keeps fresh in the refrigerator for up to one week. Keep it covered with water, and change the water every other day. Always wash tofu in cold water and drain in a colander before using.

If you are going to marinate it for grilling or baking, it is important to press it before cooking. Wash the tofu and place it on a cutting board or a flat surface with one end raised a couple of inches. Place the lower end of the board toward the sink to let the water drain off. Cover the tofu with another cutting board or a cookie sheet, and weigh it down with something heavy. Let the tofu press this way for an hour. This will eliminate the excess water and allow the tofu to absorb the marinade.

How to Prepare Vegetables: Unless specified in the recipes, don't peel vegetables. Most of the nutrients are found in the skins. Use a brush to scrub them clean.

How to Steam Vegetables: Be careful not to overcook vegetables. To retain their nutrients, steam or quickly sauté them. The steaming liquid can be saved for soup stock or added to stews and sauces.

Use a stainless-steel steamer that can be purchased in most cooking supply stores. Place the steamer in a pot with a tight-fitting lid. Pour an inch or two of water into the bottom of the pot, but not so much that it rises above the steamer. The vegetables shouldn't sit in water. Cover with a lid and cook over low heat until the vegetables are done.

How to Roast Nuts and Seeds: Roasted nuts are delicious scattered on top of a dish, served in salads, or served in small bowls to accompany your meals. Roast nuts in a dry skillet over low heat. Keep tossing them so they roast on all sides. Or roast them on a cookie sheet in a 350-degree oven for 15 minutes.

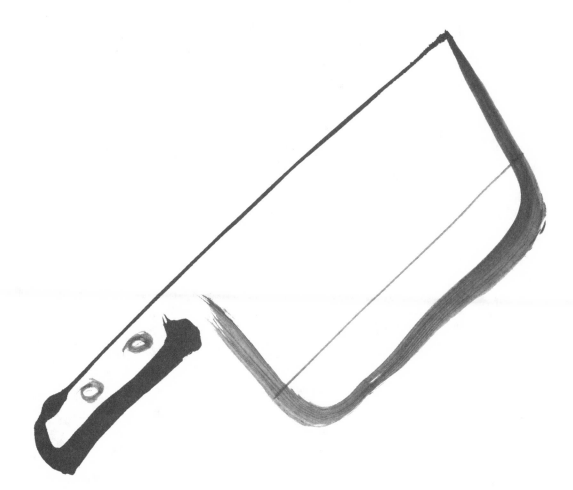

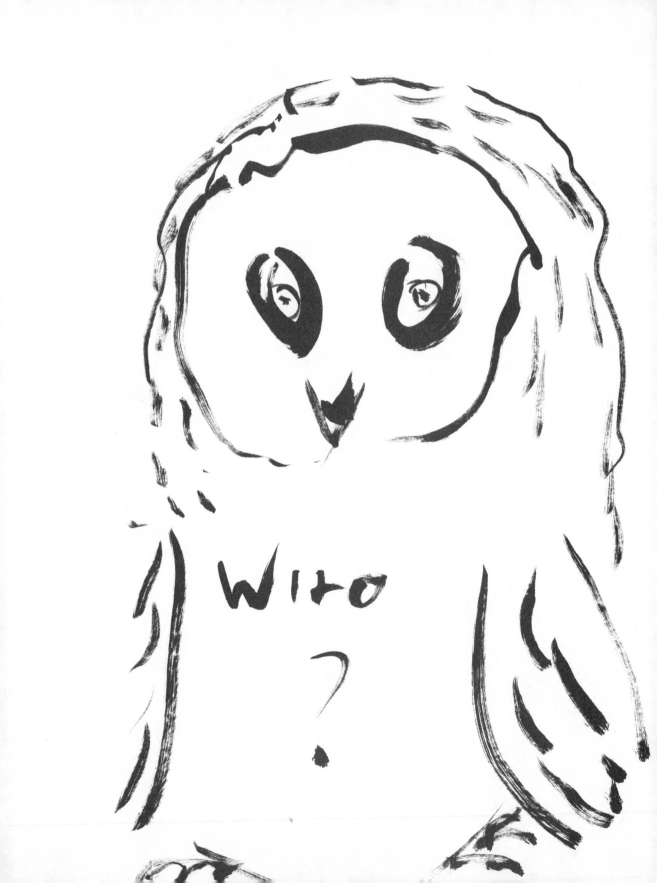

What Is the Taste of Cooking?

Before the first carrot has been peeled or onion sautéed, your sensations and experiences form the first ingredient of your cooking. And throughout the process of preparing and serving a meal, the quality of mind you bring to what you're doing has as much influence as the herbs and seasonings you use.

When Rikyu, Japan's legendary Tea master, was asked the secret of the Tea Ceremony, he replied, "Lighting the fire. Boiling the water. Whisking the tea." "Well, that seems easy to do," said the student. Rikyu responded, "If you can truly do this, then I will become your student."

To act with an undivided mind—this is the secret. Nothing is left out. Nothing extra is brought in. It sounds so simple, yet the Tea Ceremony is known to be one of Japan's most subtle and exacting art forms.

If you ask a master chef, "How do you make a wonderful soup?" he might reply, "Cut the vegetables, simmer them for an hour, and flavor to taste with seasoning."

Nothing is left out, nothing extra is brought in.

The unspoken ingredient in all cooking is the intangible spirit you bring to it. You can't buy this at the market. You can't learn it in a class or from a book, but you can let your ingredients teach you.

Look at the shapes and colors of the cabbages, carrots, zucchinis, and lettuces. Each is unique. No two eggplants are the same shade of purple. There is always a difference.

You can feel how ripe a plum or a peach is with a gentle touch. If you couldn't see, would you know just by touch the difference between an acorn squash and a tomato?

Smell the fragrance of fresh herbs and greens, and pretend you have never tasted cilantro or spinach before. How vivid your sense of taste becomes when you give it your full attention!

The zucchini, the broccoli, the asparagus, the lemon—each speaks, each has a lesson and a story to tell.

Through the medium of your senses the kitchen becomes a great workshop, a place to deepen your experience of cooking and yourself. Each chapter in this book is preceded by an essay with suggestions on how to use your time in the kitchen as an opportunity for exploration. There will also be questions that will help quiet and focus your mind, bringing you more in touch with what you do.

Some of the suggestions may appear to be extremely simple, but follow them and they may lead you to something brand new. "Things are not what they seem to be, nor are they any different." Let this paradox stated in the Lankavatara Sutra guide your journey.

You may discover that your cooking takes on a whole new flavor.

Soups

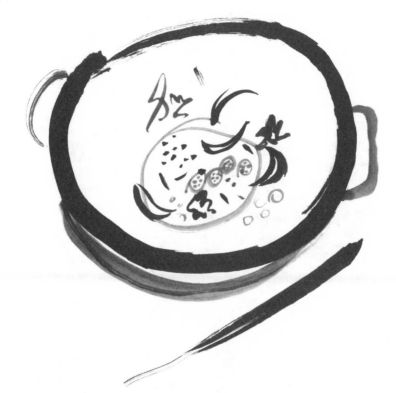

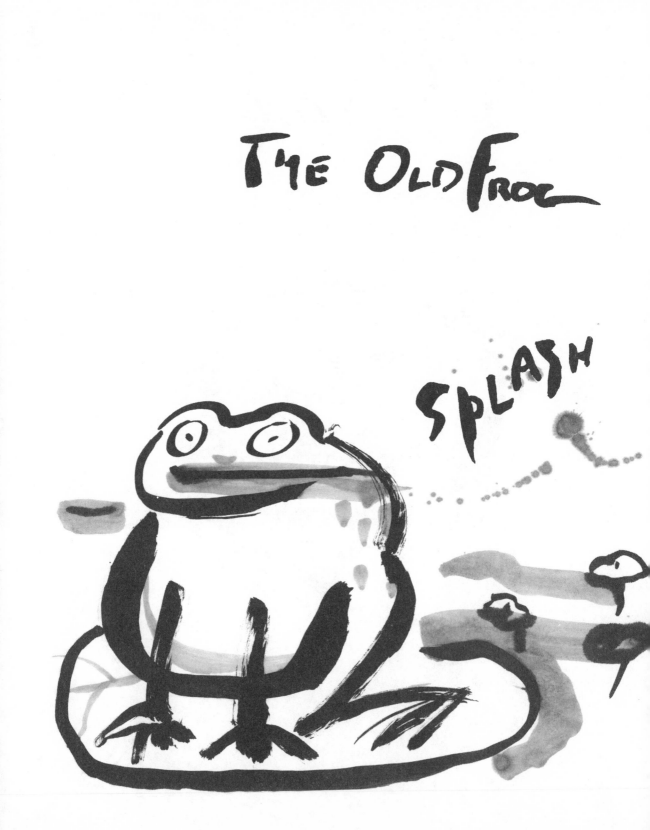

The kitchen is a kaleidoscope of shifting sights, smells, sounds, tastes, and touch. All these impressions have the power to bring us into the moment, to make us more alert to what is going on in us and around us.

> Old pond
> A frog jumps in—
> Splash
> BASHO (17TH CENTURY)

In this poem, Basho celebrates the clarity of a moment just as it is. In the kitchen there are thousands of such moments.

As cooks, we know the great delight of savoring our food. Sometimes we taste a small bite of something and chew it carefully, feeling its texture and exploring its taste.

When we smell something delicious, our mouths water. Our sense of smell helps us extract the invisible essence of things. Ginger, chili, basil, mint—we recognize these and a thousand other smells instantly.

We feel the size, shape, temperature, weight, and texture of things. Eyes closed, we can know the difference between an apple and an orange, a wooden spoon and a metal one.

Our very substance, every cell, every nerve fiber, is built to respond to the world around us. We receive the world through our senses, through the textures and aromas of life.

Soups

The secret of soups is in knowing your vegetables, and knowing what fresh herbs or spices will bring out their flavors. Most of the following soups take little time to prepare and can be made just a few hours before serving. They make excellent lunches or light dinners served with a green salad and freshly made bread.

My secret ingredient is tamari. It gives the soup its depth, as well as bringing out the intrinsic flavor of the ingredients. I rarely make soup stock, but I often use beans as the basis for soups. They thicken the soups and give them substance. Whenever you cook beans for other dishes, always reserve the liquid for a soup. It can stay refrigerated for up to 3 or 4 days.

The final touches to a bowl of soup can make a big difference in its look and taste. Garnishes such as fresh basil, parsley, mint, and feathery leaves of fennel give a spark of taste. A light dusting of Parmesan cheese or a few croutons enrich and enliven simple soups.

Carrot Soup

Pick the sweetest carrots you can find for this soup. Carrots with leafy tops are usually the freshest and best. This cream soup has a lovely orange color and is perfect to serve in any season with its refreshing tastes of lemon and cilantro. Serve it chilled in the summer with a garnish of sour cream or yogurt.

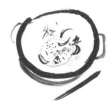

Heat the oil in a heavy-bottomed soup pot. Add the onion and garlic, and cook over high heat for 3 or 4 minutes, stirring frequently. Add the basil and carrots, and continue to cook for 5 minutes. Add the water, cover the pot with a lid, reduce the heat, and simmer until the carrots are soft, 30 to 40 minutes.

In a food processor, blend the carrots and cooking liquid until smooth. Return the soup to the stove. Add the lemon juice, tamari, and pepper to taste. Stir in the cilantro and the chili pepper. Simmer on low heat for 10 minutes. Garnish with chopped parsley or cilantro and serve immediately. If serving cold, transfer to a bowl, cover, and refrigerate for at least 4 hours.

Variation: Instead of flavoring the soup with cilantro, lemon, and chili pepper, substitute 3 tablespoons of juice from freshly grated ginger or ½ cup of fresh orange juice.

3 tablespoons olive oil

1 ½ cups chopped yellow onion

3 large garlic cloves, chopped

1 tablespoon dried basil or ¼ cup chopped fresh

1 pound carrots, sliced thinly (about 8 cups)

5 cups water

Juice of ½ lemon

1 tablespoon tamari

Freshly ground pepper

2 tablespoons chopped fresh cilantro

1 Anaheim chili pepper, minced

Finely chopped fresh parsley or cilantro for garnish

SERVES 4

Cream of Broccoli Soup

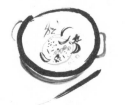

1 bunch broccoli (about 1 pound)

3 tablespoons olive oil

3 large garlic cloves, minced

1 1/2 cups chopped yellow onion

Large pinch of dried thyme

1 tablespoon dried basil

1 tablespoon mustard seeds

5 cups water

Juice of 1/2 lemon, or more to taste

Salt

Freshly ground pepper

SERVES 4 TO 6

Pale green and creamy, this is a fragrant and simply flavored soup, tangy with mustard and lemon. Broccoli is one of the most nutritious vegetables we can eat, and this soup is rich with vitamins and minerals.

Divide the broccoli into florets of equal size, 2 to 3 inches long. Trim the stalks by cutting off the ends and peeling the thick skin with a paring knife. Slice the stems into bite-size pieces. Set aside 1 cup of broccoli florets, and cut them into bite-size pieces.

Heat the oil in a medium-size soup pot, add the garlic and onion, and cook over high heat, stirring frequently, for 3 to 4 minutes, until the onion is translucent. Stir in the herbs and mustard seeds. Continue to cook for 1 minute, then toss in the broccoli (reserving the 1 cup of florets) and cook for 2 to 3 minutes, stirring continually. Add the water and bring to a simmer. Cover the pot with a lid and cook for 1 hour.

In a food processor, blend the soup to a creamy consistency. Thin it with more water if needed. Return to the stove and stir in the remaining broccoli florets. Add the lemon juice, salt, and freshly ground pepper to taste. Cook over low heat until the broccoli florets are bright green, tender, yet still crunchy, about 5 minutes. Remove from the heat and serve.

Butternut Squash and Ginger Soup

This soup, with its deep amber color and bright fragrance, is perfect for warming the heart on gray chilly days. It's light, satisfying, and easy to make.

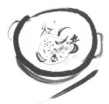

Heat the oil in a heavy-bottomed soup pot. Add the garlic and onions and cook over high heat for 3 or 4 minutes, stirring frequently, until the onions become translucent. Add the coriander, cinnamon, and the squash. Continue to cook for 5 minutes over high heat. Add the water, cover with a lid, reduce the heat, and simmer for 1 hour.

Peel the fresh ginger. Finely grate it, and then either in a towel or using your fingers, squeeze the ginger into a small cup until you have 4 tablespoons of juice.

In a food processor, blend the soup, ginger, and tamari until completely smooth. Return to the pot and cook another 5 minutes. Season to taste with salt and freshly ground pepper. A garnish of fresh cilantro really adds the final touch, and brings out all the flavors of this soup.

3 tablespoons olive oil

4 garlic cloves, chopped

1 1/2 cups chopped yellow onion

1 teaspoon ground coriander

1/4 teaspoon ground cinnamon

4 cups peeled and thinly sliced butternut squash (about a 2-pound squash)

4 cups water

1 5-inch piece fresh ginger

1 tablespoon tamari

Salt

Freshly ground pepper

Fresh chopped cilantro, for garnish

SERVES 4

Spicy Pea Soup

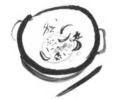

½ cup green split peas

2 tablespoons canola oil

2½ cups chopped plum tomatoes (about
   1¾ pounds)

4 scallions, sliced

1 cup bite-size-cut carrots

1½ tablespoons curry powder

5 cups water

1 tablespoon tamari

Salt

Freshly ground pepper

Finely chopped fresh parsley, for
   garnish

Sour cream, for garnish

SERVES 4

Curry spices enliven this soup and provide a wonderful contrast to the sweet carrots and tomatoes. This hearty and satisfying soup is easy to make.

Rinse the split peas, drain, and set aside.

Heat the oil in a soup pot, stir in the tomatoes, and cook over medium-high heat for 2 to 3 minutes, stirring frequently. Toss in the split peas, scallions, and carrots. Continue to cook for 5 minutes. Stir in the curry and cook for 1 minute, stirring continually. Add the water and lower the heat to simmer. Cover the pot, and cook for 1 hour.

Stir in the tamari and season to taste with salt and freshly ground pepper. Garnish with chopped parsley and a dollop of sour cream.

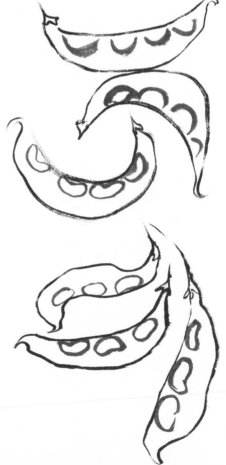

Summer Vegetable Soup with Basil Sauce

This is a great soup to make in summer when gardens are filled with luscious produce. It is a hearty meal when served with French bread and a leafy green salad.

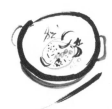

In a large soup pot, simmer the carrots, potato, onion, bay leaf, kidney beans, and tamari in the water for 1 hour.

In the meantime, prepare the basil sauce. In a food processor, blend the garlic, crushed tomatoes, basil, cheese, and olive oil to a smooth consistency. Season to taste with salt and freshly ground pepper.

Five minutes before serving, add the green beans and corn to the soup. Cook until al dente and bright green. Remove from the heat and stir in the basil sauce. Taste to adjust for seasoning. Serve garnished with chopped parsley.

½ cup diced carrots

½ cup diced red potato

½ cup finely chopped yellow onion

1 bay leaf

2 cups cooked kidney beans

3 tablespoons tamari

6 cups water

FOR THE SAUCE:

4 garlic cloves, minced

6 tablespoons tomato puree or crushed tomatoes

½ cup chopped fresh basil

½ cup grated Parmesan cheese

¼ cup virgin olive oil

Salt

Freshly ground pepper

1 cup diagonally sliced green beans

Kernels from 1 corncob

Finely chopped fresh parsley for garnish

SERVES 4

French Onion Soup

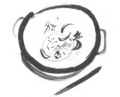

2 tablespoons olive oil

4 large garlic cloves, minced

4 cups sliced yellow onions

2 tablespoons white flour

6 cups water

4 tablespoons tamari

4 tablespoons medium dry cooking
    sherry

Salt

Freshly ground pepper

½ tablespoon olive oil

½ tablespoon butter

4 slices French bread, cut into squares
    for croutons

¾ cup grated Swiss cheese

Finely chopped fresh parsley for garnish

SERVES 4

Tamari flavoring is the secret of this easy-to-make classic. Serve it right from the broiler, with croutons and Swiss cheese melted on top.

Heat the oil in a large soup pot. Add the garlic and onions, and cook over high heat for 5 minutes, stirring frequently. Stir in the flour, reduce the heat to low, and cook for 5 more minutes. Keep stirring to keep the flour from burning. The flour absorbs the oil and makes a roux, which thickens the soup.

Stir in the water a little at a time. Partially cover with a lid and simmer for 1 hour. Ten minutes before serving, season with tamari, sherry, and salt and pepper to taste.

Heat the oil and butter in a medium-size skillet. Toss in the bread squares and sauté over medium heat until the bread is crisp and golden. Ladle the soup into crocks that can go under a broiler. Top the soup with a layer of croutons, cover lightly with cheese, and place under a hot broiler for 1 minute, until browned. Garnish with chopped parsley and serve.

Tomato and Navy Bean Soup

This soup was inspired by a rich moussaka sauce. With just a little twist here and there, it becomes an elegant soup flavored with cinnamon and clove.

Sort through the beans and discard any small stones. Rinse the beans, place in a soup pot, cover with water, and bring to a boil. Immediately drain, rinse the beans again, and place them in the pot with 4 cups water, the bay leaf, and the sage. Cover tightly with a lid and cook over low to medium heat until the beans are soft, about 1 hour.

In the meantime, heat the oil in a large skillet and sauté the garlic and onions over high heat for 3 to 4 minutes, stirring frequently. When the onions begin to look translucent, stir in the oregano, cinnamon, and clove. Lower the heat to medium and cook for 2 minutes, stirring constantly. Stir in the chopped tomatoes. Mix well and transfer to the soup pot with the beans. Cover the pot with a lid and simmer for 45 minutes, until the beans are soft. Remove the bay leaf and add the wine, tamari, and freshly ground pepper to taste. Cook for 15 minutes and serve.

1 cup dried navy beans

4 cups water

1 bay leaf

1 tablespoon dried sage

2 tablespoons olive oil

3 medium garlic cloves, minced

1 medium yellow onion, finely chopped

½ teaspoon dried oregano

1 teaspoon ground cinnamon

½ teaspoon ground clove

3 cups chopped tomatoes, canned or fresh

¼ cup red wine

1 tablespoon tamari

Freshly ground pepper

SERVES 4 TO 6

Corn Chowder

2 tablespoons canola oil

1 cup chopped yellow onion

3 garlic cloves, chopped

¾ cup chopped celery

1 ½ cups peeled and thinly sliced sweet
   potato

1 tablespoon unbleached white flour

6 cups water

3 cups fresh corn kernels

⅔ cup diced fennel bulb

2 tablespoons minced fresh cilantro

¾ cup cashews, roasted

½ cup water

¼ cup each diced red and green pepper

1 tablespoon fresh lime juice

Large pinch of cayenne

Salt

Freshly ground pepper

Fennel leaves, for garnish

SERVES 4 TO 6

The flavors of this soup are subtle with hints of cilantro, lime, and sweet fennel. Cayenne pepper tickles the palette. It's a light chowder, made with cashew milk instead of cream. It's not too rich, yet wonderfully flavorful.

Heat the oil in a large soup pot. Sauté the onions, garlic, and celery over high heat for 3 to 4 minutes, stirring frequently. When the onions begin to look translucent, add the sweet potatoes and continue to cook for 1 or 2 minutes. Lower the heat to medium and stir in the flour. Keep stirring for 5 minutes to completely cook the flour. Add the water, cover the pot with a lid, and simmer for 40 minutes.

Stir in 1 cup of the corn. Continue simmering for another 20 minutes. Blend the hot soup in a food processor until creamy and return to the pot. Add the remaining corn, the fennel, and the cilantro. Partially cover with a lid and simmer for 15 to 20 minutes.

In a meantime, roast the cashews in a dry skillet over medium heat. Stir them continually to prevent burning. In a food processor, blend the cashews with the ½ cup water until smooth.

Dice the green and red peppers the same size as the corn kernels. Stir them into the soup 5 minutes before serving. Season with lime juice and a large pinch of cayenne to taste. Stir in the cashew mixture. Season to taste with salt and freshly ground pepper. Remove from the heat and serve garnished with the feathery leaves of fennel.

Black Bean Soup

Black beans have a wonderful earthy taste that goes well with lots of garlic. The secret of this soup is the fresh cilantro and herbs.

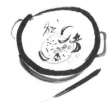

Sort through the beans and rinse them. Cover with water, bring to a boil, drain, and rinse them again. Combine the beans in a large soup pot with the water and bay leaves. Cover with a lid and simmer for 2 hours, until soft.

In a small dry skillet, toast the cumin, coriander, and oregano over low heat for 2 to 3 minutes. When the fragrance becomes strong, remove from the heat and set aside. In a separate pan, heat the oil and sauté the garlic and onions over high heat. When the onions begin to soften, stir in the thyme and the toasted herbs. Cook for a minute and add the tomato paste. Lower the heat and continue to cook for another minute or two.

Stir the tomato sauce into the pot of beans; add the cilantro. Cover with the lid and simmer on low heat for an hour.

Remove the cilantro. Stir in the chili peppers and continue cooking until the beans are soft, another 15 or 20 minutes. In a food processor, blend the beans and the bean liquid until smooth. Return to the soup pot and season to taste with tamari and freshly ground pepper. Serve garnished with chopped cilantro and a dollop of sour cream.

1 1/2 cups dried black beans

8 1/2 cups water

2 bay leaves

1 teaspoon ground cumin seeds

1 teaspoon ground coriander

1/4 teaspoon dried oregano

2 tablespoons canola oil

4 medium garlic cloves, chopped

1 large yellow onion, chopped

1 teaspoon dried thyme

1/2 cup tomato paste

*1 bunch fresh cilantro (about 2 cups),
    stems tied together*

*2 jalapeño chili peppers, minced, or 1/4
    teaspoon crushed red chili pepper*

3 tablespoons tamari

Freshly ground pepper

Chopped cilantro, for garnish

Sour cream, for garnish

SERVES 4 TO 6

Miso Soup

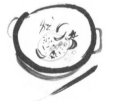

4 cups water

½ cup yellow or white miso

1 tablespoon tamari

Toasted sesame seeds, for garnish

Scallions, sliced paper thin, for garnish

Options: sautéed mushrooms, grated
   carrots, tofu

SERVES 4

Miso soup is a delicious thin broth, rich in protein. It takes about five minutes to make, so it's perfect for a quick lunch. Of the different misos available, I recommend the yellow or white variety. They are the mildest and the sweetest.

Bring the water to just below simmer. In a small mixing bowl, dissolve the miso with ½ cup of the hot water. Stir into the soup pot and mix well with the water. It is very important that the miso never boils. Flavor with tamari. Garnish with toasted sesame seeds or sliced scallions and serve.

Variations: If you want a more varied soup, add some mushrooms sautéed with a tiny bit of butter and parsley, or some thinly grated carrots tossed in at the last minute. Cut tofu into bite-size cubes and simmer in the broth before serving.

Dashi is a Japanese broth that is delicately flavored with shiitake mushrooms and kombu, a kind of seaweed. It's traditionally served with soba noodles and bowls of condiments: thinly sliced scallions, toasted nori cut into strips, roasted sesame seeds, and wasabi, a horseradish paste.

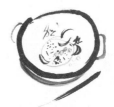

In a soup pot, bring the kombu, shiitake, and water to a boil. Lower the heat and simmer for 45 minutes.

Remove the mushrooms and kombu from the broth. Discard the stems of the mushrooms and slice the caps into small pieces. Finely chop ¼ cup of kombu and return both to the broth. Flavor the dashi with mirin, tamari, and sake. Simmer for 2 to 3 minutes and remove from the heat.

To make the condiments, toast the nori by holding it over an open flame for 1 minute, turning it frequently. Cut it into thin strips with a scissors or tear it with your hands. Toast the sesame seeds in a dry skillet over medium heat, shaking the pan or stirring the seeds so they toast on all sides. Place these in small bowls. Mix the wasabi powder with just enough water (about 1 tablespoon) to make a thick paste. Form the paste into a mound and place on a small dish.

Serve the dashi in very large soup bowls, leaving enough room for the noodles. Serve the noodles separately in a large serving bowl or put them right in with the soup. Pass around the condiments.

1 kombu, 5 to 6 inches long

3 dried or fresh shiitake mushrooms

8 cups water

2 tablespoons mirin

2½ tablespoons tamari

2 tablespoons sake

3 sheets nori

¾ cup sesame seeds

¾ cup sliced scallions

3 tablespoons wasabi powder

8 ounces cooked soba or udon noodles

SERVES 4 TO 6

White Gazpacho

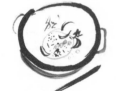

4 large cucumbers

2 ripe avocados

3 medium garlic cloves, minced

2 poblano chili peppers or 2 medium
   green bell peppers, chopped

4 scallions, chopped

2 cups water

Juice of 1½ lemons

4 tablespoons chopped cilantro

Salt

Freshly ground pepper

Pinch of cayenne

Chopped cilantro

Paprika

SERVES 4 TO 6

This soup combines the richness of avocado with the refreshing taste of cucumber. It's a cool and elegant first course for summer meals, and it is easy and quick to make. If your market carries an assortment of green chilis, try either the poblano or Anaheim chili instead of the green pepper. These are not hot chilis, but they will give the soup more zest.

Peel the cucumbers and cut in half lengthwise. Scoop out all the seeds with a spoon. Chop into large pieces and put in a blender or food processor. Cut the avocados in half and, using a spoon, scoop the avocado into the blender. Add the garlic, chopped peppers, and scallions. Blend until smooth and creamy, adding the water a little at a time. Add the lemon juice, cilantro, salt, pepper, and cayenne to taste. Serve garnished with chopped cilantro and paprika sprinkled on top.

Sweet Potato Vichyssoise

This soup is so easy to make that I often think some important ingredient must be missing. It's delicious with just the lime juice and cilantro providing a distinct contrast to the sweetness of the potatoes.

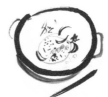

In a medium-size soup pot, heat the oil over high heat and sauté the leeks for 2 to 3 minutes. When they begin to look translucent, stir in the sweet potatoes and cook for a minute or two, stirring frequently. Add the water and bring to a simmer. Set aside enough cilantro for a garnish, and tie the bunch with a string or wrap in cheesecloth. Place in the soup pot, cover with a lid, and simmer for 45 minutes, until the potatoes are soft.

Remove the cilantro and discard. In a food processor, blend the soup until smooth and creamy. Season to taste with lime juice, salt, and freshly ground pepper. Serve garnished with chopped cilantro. To serve cold, cool to room temperature, cover, and refrigerate for at least 3 hours.

2 tablespoons olive oil

1 cup thinly sliced white of leek

3 pounds sweet potatoes, peeled and sliced 1/4 inch thick

4 cups water

1 bunch fresh cilantro (about 2 cups)

Juice of 1 1/2 limes

Salt

Freshly ground pepper

SERVES 4 TO 6

Hearty Beet Soup

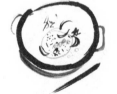

1 tablespoon canola oil

3 garlic cloves, minced

1 medium yellow onion, chopped

2 tablespoons dried basil

2 medium carrots, thinly sliced

6 medium beets (about 1 ½ pounds),
    peeled and sliced into bite-size pieces

½ pound new red potatoes, cubed

4 cups water

1 tablespoon tamari

Freshly ground pepper

Sour cream

Finely chopped fresh parsley, for
    garnish

SERVES 4 TO 6

This is a hearty and rich soup to serve in the late fall or winter. It makes a wonderful lunch served with a spinach salad and fresh hot bread. Garnish it with a swirl of sour cream or yogurt.

Heat the oil in a large soup pot. Add the garlic and onions and cook over high heat for 3 to 4 minutes, stirring frequently. When the onions look translucent, add the basil, carrots, and beets. Cook for 5 to 10 minutes to sear the ingredients. If the vegetables stick to the pot, add a tiny bit of water. Stir in the potatoes, cook for a minute or two, then add the water. Partially cover with a lid and simmer for an hour or more, until the vegetables are soft.

Remove from the stove and blend half of the ingredients in a food processor. Return to the soup pot. Flavor with tamari and freshly ground pepper to taste. Serve garnished with a dollop of sour cream and chopped parsley.

Lentil Soup with Mint

Lentils are so hearty that it is often hard to make a light and aromatic soup. Here is one that is fresh tasting, with mint and lemony flavors.

Rinse the lentils and set aside to drain.

Heat the oil in a large soup pot. Add the garlic and leeks; cook over high heat for 3 to 4 minutes. Stir in the herbs and parsnips. Continue to sauté for 5 minutes, stirring frequently. Toss in the lentils and cook another minute or so. Add the water. Bring to a simmer, stir in the tomatoes, and partially cover with a lid. Simmer for 1 hour.

Add the spinach, 2 tablespoons mint, lemon juice, and wine. Cook for 5 minutes and remove from the heat just when the spinach becomes bright green. Season to taste with tamari and freshly ground pepper. Garnish with the remaining minced mint.

¾ cup dried lentils

1 tablespoon olive oil

4 medium garlic cloves, minced

1 cup finely chopped leeks

1 teaspoon dried thyme

1 teaspoon dried sage

½ cup diced parsnips

8 cups water

1 cup finely chopped fresh or canned
plum tomatoes

1 cup finely chopped spinach

3 tablespoons minced fresh mint

2 tablespoons fresh lemon juice

2 tablespoons red wine

1 to 2 tablespoons tamari

Freshly ground pepper

SERVES 4 TO 6

Soup Stock

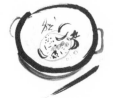

7 cups water

2 small carrots, ends trimmed

1/2 cup parsley stems

4 or 5 stems shiitake mushrooms

1 piece of celery

1/2 cup sliced leeks or yellow onions

MAKES 6 CUPS

This is a light stock perfect for delicate soups and for cooking risottos and couscous. When cooking with shiitake mushrooms, always save the stems for this stock. They add a wonderful rich flavor.

Place all the ingredients in a large pot and simmer for 1 hour, partially covered with a lid. Strain the stock and use immediately, or refrigerate up to 3 days.

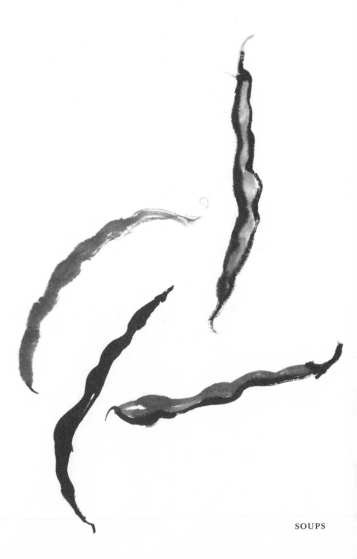

Pasta and Grains

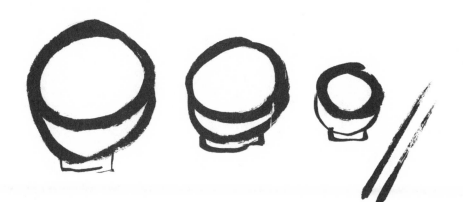

TASTE
WHAT IS
SWEET IS SWEET
WHAT IS
BITTER IS
BITTER

Cooks are connoisseurs of taste. We constantly dip our spoons into what we cook to adjust seasonings or test the flavors of a broth.

But while it's easy to savor a spoonful of soup as it cooks, we often eat with great haste when we sit down to dinner. The tastes come and go very quickly. We take a bite or two of our meal, and our thoughts wander.

When you sit down to your meal, take a moment to appreciate how it has been prepared, even if you have cooked it yourself. Notice the shapes of the vegetables, the color of the sauce, the freshness of the salad.

How do the smells of the food come to you: the aroma of fresh rosemary in the roasted potatoes, the fragrance of curry spices in the stew, the sweetness of baked apples in a pie?

As you pick up the silverware, feel the way your hand holds the fork or knife. Become aware of the movement of your arm as it brings the food to your mouth.

Take a small bite and place it on the tip of your tongue. Don't chew it. Just let it settle there for a moment or two. What is the first thing you notice? What can you taste?

Our taste buds distinguish salty, sour, bitter, or sweet sensations in different places on our tongue. Where do you taste the tartness of lemon? The bite of a hot chili pepper? The sweetness of honey?

What happens when you begin to slowly chew your food? Do you notice a whole range of tastes and textures?

What can you feel of the inside of your mouth or your teeth? Are you aware of *different sounds as you bite into an apple, swallow a sip of wine, or chew a crisp tostada?*

Even the simplest meal becomes enjoyable when it is received this way. Flavors become richer, colors seem more vibrant, smells are more alive. There is an entire world to explore even in one sip of tea or a single bite of orange. When we taste this way we open to the possibility that all of life can be savored: the fragrance of wind in the springtime, the warmth of afternoon sunshine, the whisper of a kettle boiling on the stove.

Pasta and Grains

The most delicious food is always made with the freshest ingredients, and pasta is no exception. Even if you don't make your own, there are many fresh varieties to choose from in the markets. The choices range from simple spaghetti to such elaborate and colorful pasta as red pepper fettuccine, spinach fettuccine, herb linguine, spinach cheese tortellini, Italian herb ravioli, spicy garden agnolettis, and red pepper angel hair pasta.

I cook most often with Japanese soba and udon noodles. Made from buckwheat and wheat flours, they are excellent sources of nutrition. Soba noodles are my favorite. They have a delicious nutty flavor, and are fast cooking and versatile.

Stir-fried rice and vegetables is a staple of my cooking, and I never get tired of it. It's fast and easy, and there is an endless variety of seasonal vegetables and fresh herbs that keep making it always new and interesting. Serve the rice with beans or tofu, and you have a simple nutritious meal that is completely satisfying.

For variety, make elegant rice risottos or cook polenta and grill it with fresh basil and tomatoes. Couscous pilafs with chick-peas and curry satisfy an adventurous taste.

Some Simple Pasta Ideas

Cold Soba Noodles. Refreshing to serve on hot summer days, these noodles can be cooked in advance, rinsed under cold water, drained, and chilled in the refrigerator. Serve them topped with a generous amount of East West Salsa (page 169) or toss with Orange Raspberry Vinaigrette (page 167) and top with toasted walnuts.

Spaghetti with Tomato Sauce. The recipe for the sauce is on page 161. Be inventive with this basic dish. Add some zucchini, mushrooms, or tofu to the sauce while it is cooking.

Udon Noodles with Pesto. Everyone has a favorite pesto recipe. Cook the udon noodles in boiling water until al dente. Drain and toss with the pesto. The noodles are a coffee color, so garnish with something bright like thin strips of snow peas or finely sliced red peppers.

Pasta with Cashew Ginger Sauce. This sauce is especially good with soba noodles and stir-fried tofu. For color, steam some broccoli florets until bright green. Add to the noodles at the last minute before tossing with the sauce. Garnish with thin slices of purple cabbage.

Szechuan Green Beans and Soba

This is a dish for people who love spicy food. Serve with a green salad tossed with Ewa's Honey Mustard Dressing (page 166) and grilled tofu.

Bring a large pot of water to boil, add a tiny bit of canola oil, and cook the soba until al dente, about 5 minutes. Drain and rinse under cold water. Set aside.

Wash the beans and trim the ends. Cut them diagonally into bite-size pieces. Heat the sesame oil in a large sauté pan or wok over high heat. Add the garlic and immediately stir in the green beans and red chili pepper. Lower the heat to medium and cook for 5 minutes, stirring frequently, until the beans become tender and bright green.

Add the noodles to the green beans and toss well. Season with tamari and remove from the heat. Serve sprinkled with the toasted sesame seeds.

Canola oil

12 ounces soba noodles

1 pound green beans

3 tablespoons sesame oil

3 medium garlic cloves, minced

1/2 teaspoon crushed red chili pepper

1 1/2 tablespoons tamari

1/4 cup toasted sesame seeds

SERVES 4

Pasta with Steamed Vegetables and Garlic Sauce

2 medium carrots, sliced ¼ inch thick
    on the diagonal

1 ½ cups cauliflower florets, broken in
    tiny pieces

1 ½ cups broccoli florets, broken in tiny
    pieces

12 ounces spaghetti

4 tablespoons olive oil

5 medium garlic cloves, minced

Pinch of crushed red chili pepper

1 tablespoon tamari

Freshly ground pepper

Finely chopped fresh parsley, for
    garnish

SERVES 4 TO 6

Nothing could be simpler than steaming two or three of your favorite vegetables and tossing them with spaghetti in a zesty garlic sauce. A pinch of chili pepper adds the finishing touch.

Place a metal steamer in a large pot and add 1 to 2 cups of water to just below the level of the steamer. Place the carrots in the bottom of the steamer, cover with a tight lid, and steam for 5 minutes. Add the cauliflower and, after 5 minutes, add the broccoli. Continue to steam for 3 to 4 minutes, until the broccoli is bright green, tender, yet still crunchy. Immediately rinse the vegetables under cold water. Drain and set aside.

Bring a large pot of water to a boil. Add a small amount of oil and cook the spaghetti until al dente, about 8 minutes. Drain and set aside.

Heat the olive oil in a large, heavy-bottomed pot. Add the garlic and pinch of chili pepper. Cook for a few seconds over medium heat. Immediately toss in the steamed vegetables and spaghetti. Lower the heat, cook for a minute or two, remove from the heat, and season with tamari and freshly ground pepper to taste. Serve garnished with fresh parsley.

Rigatoni with Japanese Eggplants and Basil

Rigatoni baked with the freshest summer ingredients—fresh basil, eggplants, and tomatoes—is a quick and easy casserole to make. The results are splendid.

Trim the eggplants and slice them into ⅓-inch-thick rounds. Salt them lightly and let drain in a colander for 30 minutes. Rinse well and pat dry.

Add the sliced eggplant to the tomato sauce and simmer over medium heat for 15 minutes.

Bring a large pot of water to a boil. Add a small amount of oil to the water and cook the rigatoni until al dente, 8 to 10 minutes. Drain and set aside.

In a large mixing bowl, combine the ricotta, basil, and tamari. Season with salt and freshly ground pepper to taste. It should be strongly seasoned. Gently stir in the cooked rigatoni and mix well.

Preheat the oven to 350 degrees. Ladle half the tomato sauce into the bottom of a 2-quart casserole dish. Layer all the rigatoni on top, then top with the rest of the tomato sauce. Sprinkle lightly with Parmesan cheese and bake for 35 minutes.

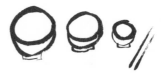

4 medium Japanese eggplants (about 1 pound)

4 cups Basic Tomato Sauce (page 161)

10 ounces cooked rigatoni

16 ounces ricotta cheese

1 cup chopped fresh basil

2 tablespoons tamari

Salt

Freshly ground pepper

½ cup grated Parmesan cheese

SERVES 4 TO 6

Noodles with Diablo Sauce and Greens

Diablo sauce is a great favorite in Mexico, where it is served on grilled fish. It's delicious with soba noodles topped with cooked beet greens and spinach. The vibrancy of the greens, the toasty flavor of the sobas, and the spicy sauce make a delightful meal.

When making the sauce, be particularly careful with the hot red chili peppers. Everyone's palate is different. You may like more or less honey and lime juice, so be prudent with these ingredients and add a bit at a time, tasting as you go.

In a food processor, blend the tomatoes, garlic, ginger juice, parsley, honey, lime juice, and sesame oil together until smooth. Taste. Add $1/8$ teaspoon chili pepper. Blend, taste, and add more pepper if you like. Season with salt.

Wash the greens to remove any sand and dirt. Heat the olive oil in a large sauté pan, add the onion, and cook over high heat for 2 to 3 minutes. Stir in the greens and cook for 5 minutes, until tender.

In the meantime, bring a large pot of water to a boil, add a tiny bit of oil, and cook the noodles until al dente, about 5 minutes. Remove from the heat and drain. Place the noodles on individual serving plates. Spoon some sauce on the noodles, place the greens on top, and spoon a topping of sauce on the greens. Be decorative. The sauce will warm up from the heat of the greens and noodles.

FOR THE SAUCE:

2 cups canned crushed tomatoes

3 large garlic cloves, chopped

3 tablespoons ginger juice, from a 3-inch piece of fresh ginger (see page 7)

1/4 cup chopped fresh parsley

2 tablespoons honey

Juice of 1 small lime

1/2 cup sesame oil

1/4 teaspoon crushed red chili pepper

Salt

3 cups chopped spinach

3 cups chopped beet greens

1 tablespoon olive oil

1/2 red onion, chopped

12 ounces soba noodles

SERVES 4

Spinach Broccoli Lasagne

This is a delicious version of lasagne, one that is light on cheese and eggs. The secret is in the sauce and the "mock ricotta."

Carefully wash the spinach. Discard the stems and coarsely chop the leaves. Rinse the tofu in cold water and set aside to drain in a colander.

Heat the oil in a large pot. Add the garlic, then the spinach and broccoli. Cook over high heat for about 10 minutes, stirring frequently, until the broccoli is half cooked. Remove from the heat and set aside.

In a large mixing bowl, mash the tofu with a fork or potato masher. Season with the tamari, nutmeg, and freshly ground pepper. Stir in ½ cup Parmesan cheese, the cooked spinach, and the broccoli. In a separate bowl, mix the eggs, then combine with the rest of the ingredients.

Bring a large pot of water to a boil. Add a small amount of oil and cook the lasagne until al dente, about 5 minutes. Since the pasta will be baked, it's important not to overcook it. Drain and rinse with cold water. Separate the lasagne so it doesn't stick together.

Preheat the oven to 350 degrees. Layer a third of the tomato sauce over the bottom of a 9 × 13-inch baking dish. Arrange one-third of the pasta over the sauce and spread one-half of the "ricotta" mix on top. For the next layer: pasta, one-third of the sauce, the rest of the "ricotta" mix. Finish with a layer of pasta and the rest of the sauce. Top with the remaining 1 cup Parmesan cheese and bake for 1 hour. Remove from the oven and cool for 10 minutes before serving.

Variations: Include other vegetables with the spinach or instead of the spinach. Onions, garlic, mushrooms, zucchini, and red pepper make a delicious filling. Sauté them as you would the spinach, but make sure you cook them al dente, as they bake for an hour.

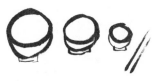

1 pound spinach

16 ounces soft tofu

1 tablespoon olive oil

4 garlic cloves, minced

1½ cups chopped broccoli

3 tablespoons tamari

½ teaspoon nutmeg

Freshly ground pepper

1½ cups freshly grated Parmesan cheese

2 eggs

¾ pound fresh spinach lasagne

4 cups Basic Tomato Sauce (page 161)

SERVES 4 TO 6

Tomato and Zucchini Primavera

12 ounces soba noodles

3 tablespoons olive oil

3 garlic cloves, minced

4 medium zucchini, sliced ½ inch thick

1 pound cherry tomatoes, cut in half

2 tablespoons chopped fresh lovage

½ cup chopped fresh basil leaves

1 tablespoon tamari

Freshly ground pepper

Finely chopped fresh parsley, for
    garnish

SERVES 4 TO 6

If you are looking for a pasta dish that requires almost no cooking time, try this primavera. Make it in the summer when the tomatoes and zucchini are tastiest. The tamari, garlic, and fresh herbs make a savory sauce. If you can't find lovage, substitute another fresh herb.

Bring a large pot of water to a boil, add a tiny bit of oil, and cook the soba until al dente, about 5 minutes. Drain, rinse under cold water, and set aside.

Heat the oil in a large heavy-bottomed pot. Add the garlic and zucchini and cook over high heat for 5 minutes, stirring frequently. When the zucchini is almost done, stir in the tomatoes, lovage, and basil. Cook for 1 minute.

If the noodles have stuck together, rinse them quickly in hot water and drain. Reduce the heat, add the noodles, and toss well. Season to taste with tamari and freshly ground pepper. Serve garnished with freshly chopped parsley.

Variations: Instead of tomatoes and zucchini, substitute Japanese eggplants sliced into thin rounds or acorn squash cut into half-moon shapes.

Mushroom Stroganoff

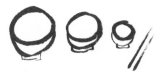

Mushrooms are the stars of this elegant pasta dish. They release their flavor into a balsamic vinegar and garlic broth, which then combines with cashews and ginger to create a luscious dish. If you make the cashew sauce in advance, the preparation time will be only thirty minutes. Many markets now carry fresh shiitake mushrooms year round. If you can't find the fresh ones, use dried shiitake, or imported dried porcini mushrooms.

If using dry mushrooms, soak them in water for half an hour before starting. When they are soft, squeeze them dry. Remove the stems from the mushrooms, saving them for soup stock, and finely chop the caps; you should have about 1½ cups. Rinse the tofu in cold water and set aside to drain for ½ hour in a colander before cutting into cubes.

Heat the olive oil in a large pan. Add the onions and garlic and cook over high heat for 3 or 4 minutes, stirring frequently. When the onions begin to look translucent, toss in the shiitake and cultivated mushrooms and the cubed tofu. Continue to cook over high heat for a few minutes to sear the mushrooms. Stir in the water and balsamic vinegar. Partially cover the pan with a lid, turn the heat down to low, and simmer for 20 minutes, until the mushrooms are well cooked. Five minutes before serving, stir in the Cashew Ginger Sauce and sour cream. Season with salt and pepper.

In the meantime, bring a large pot of water to a boil, add a tiny bit of oil, and cook the fettuccine until al dente, about 8 minutes. Drain and place the pasta in a serving dish. Add the mushroom sauce and gently toss. Served garnished with chopped parsley.

4 ounces fresh shiitake or 1 ½ ounces dry shiitake mushrooms

10 ounces firm tofu, cubed

2 tablespoons olive oil

1 yellow onion, chopped

3 medium garlic cloves, minced

2 cups sliced cultivated mushrooms

¼ cup water

¼ cup balsamic vinegar

2 cups Cashew Ginger Sauce (page 165)

½ cup sour cream

Salt

Freshly ground pepper

¾ pound fettuccine

Finely chopped fresh parsley, for garnish

SERVES 4

Spicy Spring Pasta

5 cups chopped mustard greens (about ¾ pound)

2 tablespoons canola oil

3 cloves garlic, minced

1 medium red onion, chopped

3 large carrots, julienned

3 teaspoons curry powder

2 tablespoons grated ginger

12 ounces spinach fettuccine

Tamari

Cayenne

SERVES 4 TO 6

Susan, the illustrator of this book, sent me this recipe. Inspired by the curry spices and mustard fields of India, Susan describes the dish as having "a real bite, and not just in the teeth!"

Wash the mustard greens. Discard the stems and coarsely chop the leaves.

Heat the oil in a large wok or sauté pan. Cook the garlic, onions, and carrots over high heat for 5 minutes, stirring frequently. Lower the heat to medium, stir in the curry powder, and cook for 1 minute. Toss in the mustard greens and grated ginger. Partially cover with a lid and cook for 5 minutes, until the greens are tender.

Meanwhile, bring a large pot of water to a boil, add a tiny bit of oil, and cook the fettuccine until al dente, about 8 minutes. Drain and toss with the mustard greens. Season to taste with tamari and cayenne.

Fettuccine with Fresh Greens

Sun-dried tomatoes and peppery watercress add zest to this nourishing and rich pasta dish.

Bring a large pot of water to a boil, add a tiny bit of oil, and cook the fettuccine until al dente, about 8 minutes. Drain and set aside. Wash the spinach, discard the stems of the larger leaves, and coarsely chop.

Heat the oil in a large wok or skillet. Cook the garlic and onion for 3 to 4 minutes, stirring frequently. Add the mushrooms and sun-dried tomatoes. Cook over medium-high heat for 5 to 8 minutes, until the mushrooms are well cooked. If they seem to be sticking to the pan, add a tablespoon of water.

Toss in the red peppers, spinach, 1½ cups watercress, and parsley. Cook for 5 minutes, then add the pasta. (If the pasta has stuck together, just rinse it with hot water and drain.) Season with the lemon juice, tamari, and cayenne. Cook for a minute or two, until the pasta is warm, and serve garnished with the remaining watercress.

12 ounces fettuccine

¾ pound spinach

4 tablespoons olive oil

3 large garlic cloves, minced

½ large red onion, chopped

8 mushrooms, sliced

*3 to 4 sun-dried tomatoes packed in
   olive oil, sliced in narrow strips*

½ red pepper, minced

2 cups loosely packed watercress leaves

½ cup chopped fresh parsley

1 tablespoon fresh lemon juice

2 tablespoons tamari

Cayenne

SERVES 4 TO 6

Red Rice Pilaf

1 cup long-grain brown rice

2 cups water

1/2 small acorn squash

1 1/2 tablespoons olive oil

1 medium red onion, chopped

1 cup chopped tomatoes

1 1/2 cups coarsely chopped spinach

3/4 cup sliced red pepper

1/4 cup finely chopped fresh basil

1 tablespoon lemon juice

1 tablespoon tamari

Freshly ground pepper

Cayenne

*1/4 cup finely chopped fresh basil or
   parsley, for garnish*

SERVES 4

Tomatoes and acorn squash make a creamy rice pilaf. If you have some leftover Tomato and Navy Bean Soup, use it instead of the fresh tomatoes. The hints of cinnamon and clove are wonderful in this pilaf.

Rinse the rice well and drain it. Put it in a heavy pot with the water, cover tightly with a lid, and bring to a boil. Immediately reduce the heat to low and simmer for 40 minutes.

In the meantime, remove the seeds from the squash, cut it into thin slices, and cut those in thirds or bite-size pieces.

Heat the oil in a large pan or wok. Sauté the onion and squash over high heat for 4 to 5 minutes, stirring frequently. When the onions begin to look translucent, stir in the tomatoes. Cook for 2 to 3 minutes. Toss in the spinach. Reduce the heat to a simmer, cover with a lid, and cook until the squash is soft, about 20 minutes. Stir in the red pepper, basil, lemon juice, and tamari. Cook another 5 minutes.

Stir in the cooked rice. Season to taste with freshly ground pepper. To make it spicy, add a pinch or two of cayenne. Garnish with fresh basil or parsley.

Risotto with Swiss Chard

Swiss chard is known as a powerhouse of nutrition. Like spinach, it enhances the look of rice dishes with its ribbons of green. This risotto is flavored with fresh herbs, which heighten the delicate sweetness of the chard.

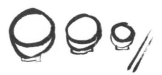

Wash the Swiss chard. Discard the stems and cut the leaves into strips. Place in a large pot, cover tightly with a lid, and cook over medium heat for 5 minutes, or until the leaves have cooked down and are tender. You don't need oil. Remove from the heat, drain in a colander, and set aside.

Heat the oil in a medium-size pot. Add the garlic, onions, and herbs. Cook over high heat for 3 to 4 minutes, stirring frequently. When the onions begin to look transparent, stir in the rice. (Do not rinse the rice beforehand. Its starch is essential for creaminess.) Cook the rice for a couple of minutes, then stir in the Swiss chard. Continue cooking over high heat for another 2 minutes.

In the meantime, bring the soup stock to a simmer. Add 2 cups of stock to the rice or enough to just cover it, reduce the heat, and let it simmer gently, stirring every once in a while. When the broth has become absorbed by the rice, add more stock to just cover. Again, let this simmer gently until it has become absorbed by the rice. Continue this process for 15 minutes, until the rice is al dente and the risotto is creamy.

Five minutes before the risotto is done, stir in the white wine. Season to taste with salt and freshly ground pepper and continue to cook 2 or 3 more minutes. Garnish with chopped parsley and serve with freshly grated Parmesan cheese on the side.

¾ pound Swiss chard

2 tablespoons olive oil

2 medium garlic cloves, minced

1 medium onion, diced

1 tablespoon minced fresh rosemary

1 tablespoon minced fresh sage

3 tablespoons finely chopped fresh parsley

2 cups Arborio rice

6 cups Soup Stock (page 32)

2 tablespoons dry white wine

Salt

Freshly ground pepper

Parmesan cheese

SERVES 4 TO 6

Asparagus Risotto

FOR THE BROTH:

4 cups water

6 to 8 parsley stems

8 mushroom stems

1 celery stalk

1 1/2 cups dry white wine

1/4 cup sliced red onion

1 teaspoon lemon juice

1 pound asparagus

2 cups Basmati or long-grain rice

2 tablespoons olive oil

3/4 cup chopped red onion

1 1/2 cups yellow squash, cut in half,
*   then sliced 1/4 inch thick*

Salt

Freshly ground pepper

Parmesan cheese

Paprika

SERVES 4

This is a delicate spring and summer dish. The rice is sautéed with onions and yellow summer squash, then simmered with asparagus in a light broth of lemon and white wine. For this risotto, the subtle flowery flavor of Basmati rice is ideal; long-grain brown rice is also good.

In a small soup pot, combine all the broth ingredients. Cover tightly with a lid and simmer for 1/2 hour before beginning the rice. Keep the broth simmering on the stove while cooking the rice.

Cut the tips from the asparagus and set aside. Trim the ends and slice the stems on the diagonal into thin 1/4-inch slices. Rinse the rice and set aside to drain.

Heat the olive oil in a medium pot. Sauté the onions and yellow squash over high heat for 3 to 4 minutes, stirring frequently. When the onions begin to look translucent, stir in the rice. Cook for 1 minute, stirring constantly.

Strain the vegetables from the broth and mix 1 1/2 cups of broth into the rice, or enough just to cover the rice. Adjust the heat to a full simmer. Partially cover the pot with a lid. Keep your eye on the rice and when it has absorbed most of the liquid, add more broth, just to cover. Continue in this way until all the broth is gone and the rice is al dente. This should take about 30 minutes.

Just before adding the last portion of broth to the rice, blanch the asparagus tips briefly in the simmering broth for a couple of minutes until bright green. Scoop them out with a slotted spoon and set aside.

Add the last bit of broth to the rice and stir in the asparagus stems. Simmer for 5 minutes. Remove from the heat. season with salt and freshly ground pepper to taste. Top with the asparagus tips and freshly grated Parmesan cheese. Sprinkle with paprika and serve.

Stir-Fry Rice and Vegetables

One of the most nutritious ways to cook vegetables is to sauté them quickly over very high heat. I use this technique more than any other. The fast cooking allows the vegetables to retain their nutrients, color, and liveliness. Cooked rice is tossed in at the last moment, and the dish is seasoned lightly with tamari.

Use a well-seasoned skillet or wok. Heat 1 or 2 tablespoons of oil over high heat and quickly toss in the vegetables. Timing is crucial here. First, add onions and such firm, longer-cooking vegetables as carrots and squashes. Thickly cut vegetables will take longer to cook than thinly sliced ones. Softer vegetables, such as red peppers and leafy greens, go into the pan last. Keep the heat quite high and keep tossing the vegetables. The East West Stir-Fry (page 52) is an excellent recipe for developing this cooking technique.

Mushrooms are good to add in the middle of cooking. If your sauté becomes dry and the vegetables begin to stick to the pan, toss in a few sliced mushrooms, cook for a minute, then add a tiny bit of water to the sauté. Even a few drops will be enough. This will cause the mushrooms to release their juices immediately.

Always cut the vegetables into beautiful shapes. Slice sweet potatoes very thin so they almost melt in the sauté, invisibly sweetening it. Add tofu or beans whenever you can. Purple cabbage will turn everything purple, so add at the last moment of cooking.

East West Stir-Fry

1 cup short-grain brown rice

2 cups water

1 tablespoon canola oil

¾ cup chopped yellow onion

2 cups sliced mushrooms

1 large red pepper, cut in bite-size strips

3 cups chopped bok choy

1 to 2 tablespoons tamari

Freshly ground pepper

SERVES 4

Use this recipe as a basis for all stir-fries. Combine vegetables with color and taste in mind. In this recipe the red peppers and bright green bok choy make it fresh and vibrant.

Wash and drain the rice. Put it in a heavy pot, add the water, cover with a tight lid, and bring to a boil. When steam escapes from the lid, immediately reduce the heat to low and simmer for 40 minutes.

Heat the oil in a large sauté pan or wok. Add the onion and cook over high heat for 3 to 4 minutes, stirring frequently. When the onion begins to look translucent, stir in the mushrooms. Cook for a minute, then add 1 teaspoon of water. The mushrooms will sizzle. Keep stirring them every so often. When they have cooked for 5 minutes, toss in the red pepper. Cook 2 or 3 minutes, then add the bok choy. Cook until the leaves become bright green, about 2 minutes. Lower the heat to medium and stir in the cooked rice. Season with tamari and freshly ground pepper. Stir for a minute or two until the rice is well mixed, then remove from the heat.

Primavera Rice

This is a particularly colorful and delicious stir-fry. It makes a satisfying one-dish meal and is fairly quick to prepare. If you don't have all the ingredients on hand, make do with what you have, although the lima beans and spinach are essential.

Wash the rice, drain, and place in a medium pot with the water. Cover with a tight lid, bring to a boil, reduce the heat to low, and simmer for 40 minutes.

Wash the spinach, discard any large stems, and chop coarsely.

Heat the oil in a large sauté pan or wok. Add the leeks and carrots, and cook over high heat for 5 minutes, stirring frequently. Stir in the zucchini, yellow squash, and mushrooms. If they begin to stick, add 1 teaspoon of water. Lower the heat to medium and cook for 2 or 3 minutes, stirring frequently. Toss in the spinach and celery. Mix well with the rest of the sauté and cover with a lid. Cook for 5 minutes.

When the spinach has cooked down, toss in the peppers and lima beans. Cook for 3 to 4 minutes. Stir in the cooked rice. Season with tamari and freshly ground pepper to taste. Continue to stir for a minute or two, until the rice is hot. Remove from the heat and serve.

1 cup long-grain brown rice

2 cups water

3/4 pound spinach

2 tablespoons canola oil

3/4 cup sliced leeks

1 carrot, sliced thin on the diagonal

1 zucchini, cut on the diagonal

2 small yellow summer squash, sliced 1/4 inch thick

4 mushrooms, sliced

2 celery ribs, thinly sliced

1/2 green bell pepper and 1/2 red bell pepper, chopped

1 cup baby lima beans

1 to 2 tablespoons tamari

Freshly ground pepper

SERVES 4

Polenta

Polenta is one of my favorite foods to cook. Although a simple, coarse cornmeal, it is extremely versatile. It can be flavored with tomatoes and fresh basil, or green chilis and red peppers. It can be baked in a casserole or grilled until crisp.

Basic Polenta

5 cups water

Pinch of salt

1 ½ cups of polenta

¾ cup grated cheddar, Monterey Jack, or Parmesan cheese

2 tablespoons butter

1 ½ tablespoons tamari

Salt

Freshly ground pepper

SERVES 4

In a large saucepan, bring the water to a boil. Add a pinch of salt and slowly whisk in the polenta so it doesn't form lumps. Lower the heat and cook for 10 minutes, stirring constantly. Stir in the cheese, butter, and tamari. Cook slowly for another 10 minutes. Season to taste with salt and freshly ground pepper.

For a soft polenta, keep it warm in the top of a double boiler over simmering water until serving.

To grill or broil polenta, follow this procedure. After you have seasoned the polenta, pour it into a 9 × 13-inch rectangular pan or a 12-inch round pan to a depth of 1 inch. Set aside to cool. In 30 minutes when firm, cut it into squares or triangles. Brush both sides with olive oil and cook on a grill or under the broiler until crisp and browned. Serve topped with Tomato Salsa (page 84) or Pesto (page 164).

Polenta with Basil and Tomatoes

This is always a favorite in summer when the tomatoes are at their finest and the basil is sweet.

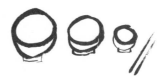

Follow the basic polenta recipe. In the last minute of cooking, stir in 1 cup chopped tomatoes and ¾ cup finely chopped fresh basil. Pour into a 12-inch pie plate or 9 × 13-inch rectangular pan. Cool and slice into quarters. Either grill it or serve it cool, arranged on a serving platter.

Polenta with Green Chilis and Red Peppers

Hot jalapeño peppers make a New Mexican version of polenta. It can be grilled or served soft alongside a black bean chili.

Basic Polenta (page 54)
¼ to ½ cup minced and seeded jalapeño chili peppers
½ red pepper

Follow the basic polenta recipe. Add the peppers when you add the cheese. For a soft polenta, keep it warm in the top of a double boiler until serving. Or pour into a 12-inch pie plate or 9 × 13-inch rectangular pan. Cool, then slice into quarters.

Polenta Casserole

This layered casserole is great served in the winter with a savory ratatouille or Sweet Red Sauce.

Basic Polenta (page 54)
4 cups Sweet Red Sauce (page 162) or Ratatouille (page 131)
½ cup grated Parmesan cheese

SERVES 4 TO 6

Make the polenta in advance. Pour into a 9 × 13-inch rectangular pan to a depth of ½ inch. Cool until firm, about 30 minutes.

Preheat the oven to 350 degrees. In the bottom of individual ovenproof plates, spread a layer of sauce or ratatouille. Cut the polenta slices to fit the shape of the plates and place on top of the sauce. Cover the polenta with the rest of the sauce, top with Parmesan cheese, and bake for 20 minutes.

A less elaborate way to make this casserole is to pour the just-cooked polenta directly into a 9-inch casserole dish. Top with the sauce. Cover with Parmesan cheese and bake for 20 minutes.

Variation: Polenta with Black Beans

This is delicious and easy to make if you have some Black Bean Chili (page 78) on hand. Prepare the Basic Polenta. Pour half the amount into a 9-inch square baking dish. Spread 2 cups Black Bean Chili on top and cover with the rest of the polenta. Top with grated cheese if you wish and bake in the oven at 350 degrees for half an hour. Serve with Tomato Salsa (page 84).

Couscous with Mushrooms

Couscous is a traditional dish enjoyed throughout North Africa. It's easy to cook and perfect to make when you have very little time to prepare dinner. It takes only five minutes. This version is rich with deep earthy flavors of mushrooms. If they are available, use such wild mushrooms as shiitakes or chanterelles. Dry porcinis or dry shiitakes are also good.

Make the stock in advance. Wash the mushrooms and pat dry. Thinly slice them.

Heat the oil and butter in a large skillet or wok, and sauté the mushrooms over medium-high heat for 10 minutes, stirring frequently. Season with lemon juice, tamari, and freshly ground pepper.

Measure the couscous into a medium-size pot with a tight-fitting lid. In a separate pot, bring the stock to a boil and stir it into the couscous. Immediately cover and let it sit for 5 minutes. Uncover and fluff the couscous with a fork. Mix in the cooked mushrooms and scallions. Taste and adjust the seasoning. Garnish with parsley and serve.

1 1/2 cups Soup Stock (page 32)

4 ounces fresh wild or cultivated mushrooms

1 tablespoon canola oil

1 tablespoon butter

1 tablespoon lemon juice

1 tablespoon tamari

Freshly ground pepper

1 1/2 cups whole wheat couscous

3 scallions, thinly sliced

Minced fresh parsley, for garnish

SERVES 4

Curry Pilaf with Chick-Peas and Couscous

1 cup whole wheat couscous

1 cup Soup Stock (page 32), at a boil

1 tablespoon olive oil

2 garlic cloves, minced

1/2 red onion, chopped

1 tablespoon curry powder

1/2 red pepper, minced

1 cup cooked chick-peas

1 cup fresh green peas

1/2 cup chopped fresh parsley

1 teaspoon tamari

Freshly ground pepper

SERVES 4

Couscous has a wonderful ability to absorb flavors. In this pilaf, the buttery taste of chick-peas combined with spicy curry makes an irresistible dish. The flavors intensify with time. If you have any left over, serve it the next day as a salad.

Measure the couscous into a pot with a tight-fitting lid. Pour the boiling stock over the couscous, cover, and let sit for 5 minutes. Fluff with a fork and set aside.

Heat the oil in a large wok or skillet and cook the garlic and onions over high heat for 3 to 4 minutes, stirring frequently. When the onions begin to look translucent, stir in the curry powder. Continue to cook for 1 minute. Add 1 tablespoon of water, the red pepper, and the chick-peas. Stir well, lower the heat to medium, and cook for 5 minutes, stirring frequently.

Stir in the green peas, parsley, and the cooked couscous. Mix well over low heat for a couple of minutes until the couscous is hot. Remove from the heat and season with tamari and freshly ground pepper.

Wild Rice Pilaf

Wild rice is not rice, but the seed of a swamp-growing grass. Before it was commercially grown, it grew wild in Minnesota, where it was harvested by hand. Serve this pilaf with baked acorn squash or roasted autumn vegetables.

Wash the rices, drain, and set aside. Heat the oil in a medium pot. Sauté the onion over high heat for 3 to 4 minutes, stirring frequently. When the onion looks translucent, stir in the rice, thyme, and marjoram. Cook for 2 or 3 minutes, stirring. Add the water and apricots, stir, and cover tightly with a lid. Bring to a boil. When steam escapes from the lid, immediately turn the heat to low. Cook for 40 minutes.

    Add the celery, squash, and red pepper to the top of the rice. Cover immediately with the lid and continue to cook 10 more minutes. This will steam the vegetables and cook them al dente.

    Remove from the heat. Fluff the rice and vegetables together with a fork. Season to taste with salt and freshly ground pepper. Garnish with chopped parsley or fennel.

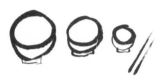

1 cup long-grain brown rice

1 cup wild rice

2 tablespoons olive oil

²/₃ cup finely chopped red onion

1 teaspoon dried thyme

1 teaspoon dried marjoram

4 cups water

¹/₂ cup chopped dried apricots

¹/₂ cup diced celery

²/₃ cup finely chopped yellow squash

¹/₂ cup finely chopped red pepper

Salt

Freshly ground pepper

*¹/₄ cup finely chopped fresh parsley or
    fennel leaves, for garnish*

SERVES 4

Curries, Mexican Tastes, Sushi Ideas, and Pizzas and Vegetable Tarts

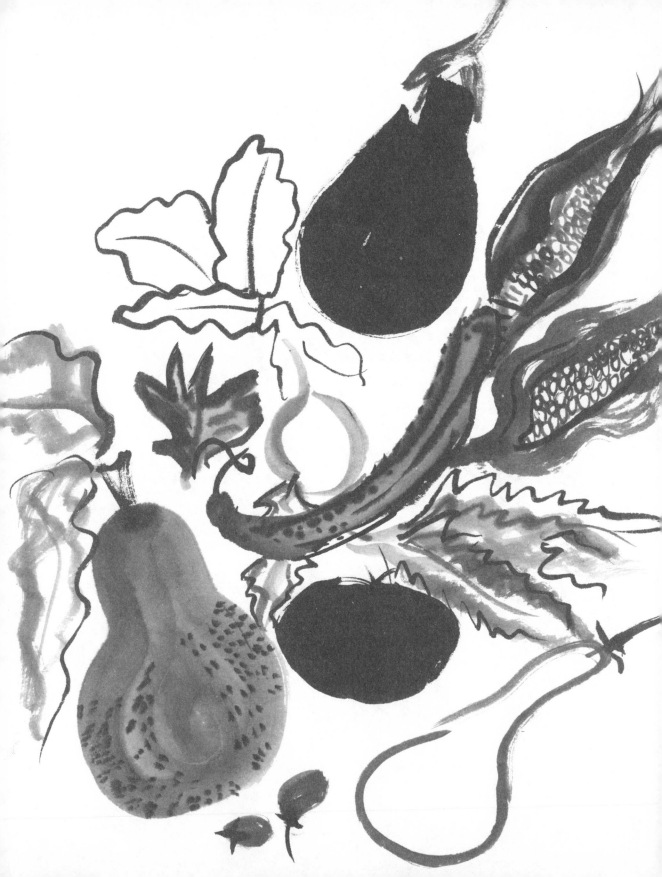

These recipes are fun to prepare and are always a good excuse to invite friends for dinner. Everyone loves a curry meal with all its mysterious spices and wonderful array of companion dishes: sweet and spicy chutneys, cool yogurt raitas, toasted cashew nuts, and rice pilafs with raisins. There are many wonderful chutneys to choose from in the markets—mango, apple nut, and cranberry ginger. In summer, when the mint is fresh, make your own apple mint chutney.

Mexican food is also a welcome treat, excellent to serve for parties or for small gatherings. Homemade refried beans wrapped in hot tortillas, freshly made spicy salsa, avocado salads, and marvelous toppings and sauces are easy to prepare. This is a festive food.

For a light dinner or lunch, sushi is perfect as an opener for soup and salad. Make it for picnics and serve it nestled in Japanese boxes. Bring along a thermos of hot water and whisk in some green tea when you're ready to eat.

Pizzas are always popular. I once made pizza for sixty people who came to Dai Bosatsu for a summer celebration. Four of my friends helped in the kitchen as we prepared fourteen pizzas, all different. It was a memorable cooking experience, and the party was a great success. We served the pizzas with corn on the cob, avocado red pepper salad, and strawberry shortcake for dessert.

Curries

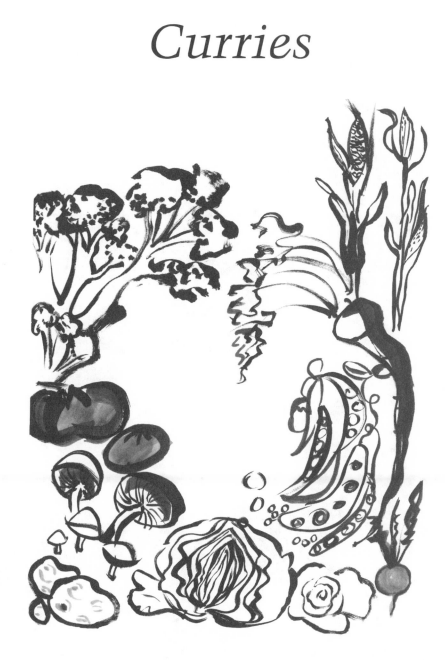

In ancient China there was a cook who was famous for his exquisite food, but even more famous for the razorlike sharpness of his knives. He used the same knives year after year, and they always kept their edge even though he never sharpened them.

The emperor heard about this amazing cook and sent for him. He was determined to find out what magic the cook used to keep his knives so sharp.

All the members of court went to watch as the cook set about preparing a sumptuous banquet for the emperor. They watched while he sliced and chopped all the vegetables. They watched carefully as he prepared Peking duck and the other exotic items on the menu—bear claws, camel humps, fish lips, and shark's-fin soup. They saw how his knives cut gracefully and easily through everything. It was as though they possessed eyes and knew exactly how to weave their way through intricate places. What was his secret?

The cook was surprised by all the attention. It seemed so simple to him. In response to all the questions he had but one simple answer: "The knife sharpens itself as it cuts."

The kitchen is a place that sharpens us. It's a place that wakes us up. Our sense of smell becomes keener. We taste with greater subtlety. We see with more clarity and our movements become quick and sure.

But there are times when we are not as sensitive, not as focused. We are distracted and nothing seems to go right. In the kitchen the results are easy to notice. The sauce burns, the bread doesn't rise, and dishes slip out of our hands.

Cooking requires that we be fully present. This is one of its greatest teachings.

It keeps bringing us back to what is happening in the moment and continually calls our attention to what we are doing.

We smell when the cake is ready to come out of the oven and we taste when the soup is almost done to perfection. When the water boils on the stove, we turn down the heat.

Through cooking we can become more responsive to what is happening around us. In the very same way that the Chinese cook was able to sharpen his knives just by using them, we can sharpen our lives by living them with awareness, moment by moment.

> "Sharpened over long years of training,
> His skill attained a cutting edge in living."

This poem was written about the great Tea master Rikyu. His art was to transform an everyday event into something exquisitely simple and deeply profound. Imagine our lives becoming transformed through making tea or cooking a meal.

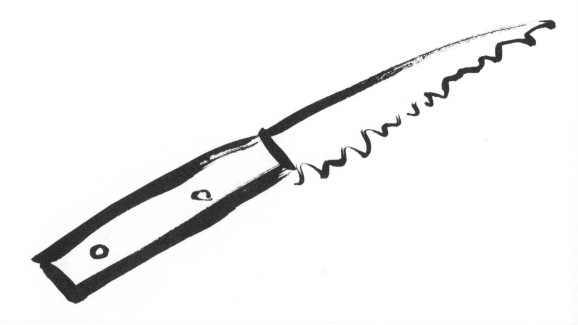

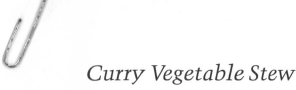

Curry Vegetable Stew

This stew is sweetened with cinnamon and cloves and although it is not a hot curry, the ginger and garlic give it a lively flavor.

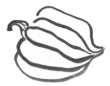

Heat the oil in a large heavy-bottomed pot or wok. Add the garlic and onions and cook over medium heat for 1 minute, then stir in the curry powder, cardamom, cloves, and cinnamon. Reduce the heat to low and cook for 2 to 3 minutes, stirring frequently, until the onions become soft. Add the carrots, squash, and potatoes. Sauté for 1 minute to seal in all the spices. Add the water and ginger. Cover and simmer for about 20 minutes, until the vegetables are soft.

Check every so often to make sure the water level just covers the ingredients; add more water if necessary. Taste the sauce after it has cooked about 10 minutes; it may need more curry or ginger. If so, now is the time to add it.

When the carrots and potatoes are soft, stir in the broccoli and string beans. Cook for 5 to 10 minutes over medium heat, until they turn bright green and are al dente. Season with tamari, salt, freshly ground pepper, and cayenne to taste. Garnish with chopped parsley or cilantro and sprinkle the roasted cashews on top.

Variations: Make this stew with other vegetables if butternut squash is not in season or potatoes aren't available. Cauliflower is a favorite in curries. Tofu is a delicious addition, since it absorbs flavors very well, and fresh green peas are traditional. For a sweeter curry, include ½ cup raisins when simmering the vegetables.

2 tablespoons canola oil

3 medium garlic cloves, minced

1 medium yellow onion, chopped

2 tablespoons curry powder

1 teaspoon ground cardamom

1 teaspoon ground cloves

1 teaspoon ground cinnamon

2 carrots, sliced bite size

*1 cup butternut squash, peeled and cut
    into ½-inch cubes*

*4 new red potatoes (about ½ pound),
    cut into ½-inch cubes*

½ cup water

2 inches ginger, peeled and finely grated

1 cup broccoli florets

2 cups trimmed and halved string beans

1 tablespoon tamari

Salt

Freshly ground pepper

Cayenne

*Finely chopped fresh parsley or cilantro,
    for garnish*

½ cup cashew nuts, roasted and chopped

SERVES 4

Coconut Curry Vegetables

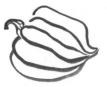

2 tablespoons canola oil

3 large garlic cloves, minced

½ medium yellow onion, sliced or
  chopped

2 large carrots, sliced ¼ inch thick on
  the diagonal

½ medium acorn squash (about ½
  pound), cut into bite-size pieces

3 teaspoons curry powder

14 ounces coconut milk

¼ teaspoon hot red chili pepper flakes

3 cups broccoli florets

2 cups fresh or frozen peas

1 tablespoon tamari

Freshly ground pepper

SERVES 4

Coconut milk, flavored with curry, makes a rich and luscious sauce for carrots, acorn squash, and broccoli. Hot chili peppers make it fiery. Serve with a nutty brown rice and an apple and fresh mint chutney.

Heat the oil in a large heavy pot. Add the garlic and onions and cook over high heat for 3 to 4 minutes, stirring frequently. When the onions begin to look translucent, toss in the carrots and acorn squash. Cook for a couple of minutes to sear the vegetables, then stir in the curry powder. Reduce the heat to medium. Continue to cook for 5 minutes. If the vegetables start to stick to the pan, add ¼ cup water.

Stir in the coconut milk and chili pepper flakes, partially cover with a lid, and simmer for about 30 minutes, until the vegetables are soft. The coconut milk will cook down to a stewlike consistency.

When the vegetables are soft, stir in the broccoli, cover, and continue to simmer for 5 minutes, until the broccoli turns a bright green and is still crunchy. Stir in the peas and season with tamari and freshly ground pepper to taste. Remove from the heat. The broccoli and peas should be a bright green, so be careful not to overcook.

Spicy Squash Stew

This is not really a curry, and it's not really a chili. It's kind of in between and one of my favorites. Serve with rice, an assortment of chutneys, roasted nuts, and sour cream on the side.

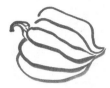

In a dry skillet, toast the almonds over medium heat for 5 minutes, until lightly browned. Set aside and use the same pan to toast the sesame seeds. Keep tossing the pan to prevent them from burning. In a food processor, grind the almonds and sesame seeds to a coarse powder.

Heat the oil in a heavy bottomed pot or large wok. Sauté the garlic and onion over high heat for 3 to 4 minutes, stirring frequently. When the onions begin to look translucent, stir in the squash, mushrooms, cumin, oregano, chili powder, and red pepper flakes. Continue to cook over medium-high heat for 5 minutes. If the vegetables begin to stick to the pan, add 1 tablespoon of water.

Add the tomatoes and just enough water to cover all the ingredients. Partially cover with a lid and simmer until the squash is soft, about 20 minutes. Taste to adjust the chili and hot pepper seasoning. If more is needed, add it now. While the vegetables are simmering, check every so often to make sure there is enough liquid covering the vegetables. If not, add more water.

When the squash is soft, stir in the ground almonds, sesame seeds, and the cauliflower. Partially cover with a lid and simmer for 10 minutes, until the cauliflower is soft. Stir in the peas and cook for 1 minute. When they turn bright green, immediately remove from the heat. Season with tamari and freshly ground pepper, and serve.

¾ cup almonds

¼ cup sesame seeds

1 tablespoon canola oil

3 large garlic cloves, minced

1 large yellow onion, chopped

1 medium butternut squash (about 1 pound), peeled and cut into ½-inch cubes

2½ cups sliced mushrooms

1½ teaspoons ground cumin

½ teaspoon dried oregano

¼ teaspoon chili powder

1 teaspoon crushed red pepper flakes

1 cup chopped tomatoes

½ cup water

2 cups cauliflower florets

2 cups fresh or frozen green peas

2 tablespoons tamari

Freshly ground pepper

SERVES 4 TO 6

Summer Mint and Apple Chutney

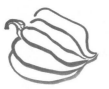

1 cup raisins

1 apple

1 orange

½ cup fresh mint

2 tablespoons fresh lemon juice

Salt

SERVES 4

Make this chutney in the summer, when fresh mint is abundant. If you like it hot and spicy, mince up a jalapeño pepper and add it to the ingredients.

At least 1 hour in advance, soak 1 cup raisins in enough water to just cover them. When they have softened, drain, saving the liquid.

Core the apple and peel the orange. Cut them in large pieces. Place all the ingredients, except the raisin liquid, into a food processor. Blend well, then add the raisin liquid a little at a time until the consistency is smooth. Season to taste with salt.

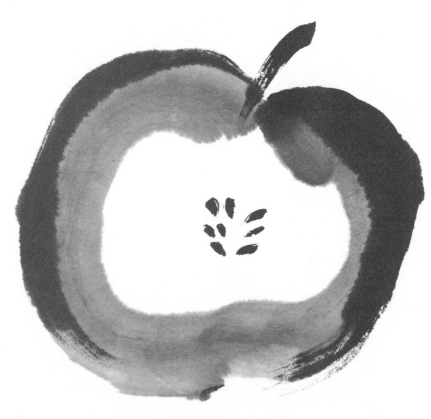

Yogurt Raita with Cucumber

Spicy and cool, this raita goes well with hot curries. It can also be served as a salad.

Mix all the ingredients together. Be careful when adding the cayenne—a little goes a long way. Chill in the refrigerator for at least 30 minutes before serving.

2 cups plain yogurt

3 medium garlic cloves, minced

2 medium cucumbers, peeled, seeded, finely chopped (about 2 ½ cups)

Salt

Cayenne

SERVES 4

Yogurt Raita with Ginger and Honey

This raita offers a sweet contrast to spicy curries. It is so delicious you can also serve it as a dessert, topped with fresh strawberries.

Peel and finely grate the ginger. Squeeze the juice from the grated ginger either in a towel or with your fingers. Mix 3 tablespoons into the yogurt and stir in the honey. Taste to adjust the flavors. Chill in the refrigerator for 1 hour before serving.

3- to 4-inch piece fresh ginger

2 cups plain yogurt

2 tablespoons honey

MAKES 2 CUPS

Tomato Coconut Raita

½ cup unsweetened shredded coconut

½ pound plum tomatoes, finely chopped

¼ cup minced poblano chili pepper or
   green bell pepper

1 cup plain yogurt

Salt

1 teaspoon canola oil

1 teaspoon mustard seeds

MAKES 3 CUPS

Here's a raita sweet with coconut and tangy with mustard and chili. It's also colorful, with specks of red and green.

In a dry skillet, toast the coconut over low heat for 5 minutes, stirring frequently to prevent burning. When it becomes golden brown, remove from the heat and toss into a mixing bowl with the tomatoes and chili pepper. Stir in the yogurt and season to taste with salt.

Heat the oil in a small pan over medium heat. Cook the mustard seeds, stirring frequently, until they begin to jump. Add the oil and seeds to the yogurt. Mix well. Chill for 1 hour before serving.

Mexican Tastes

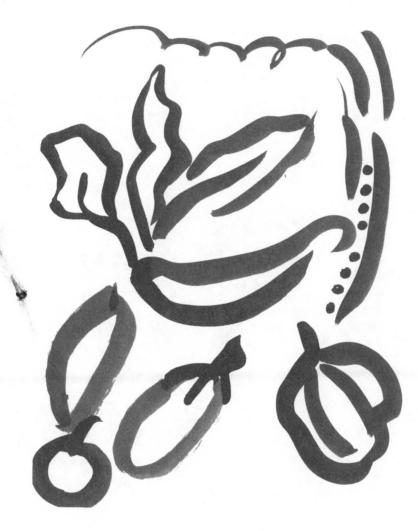

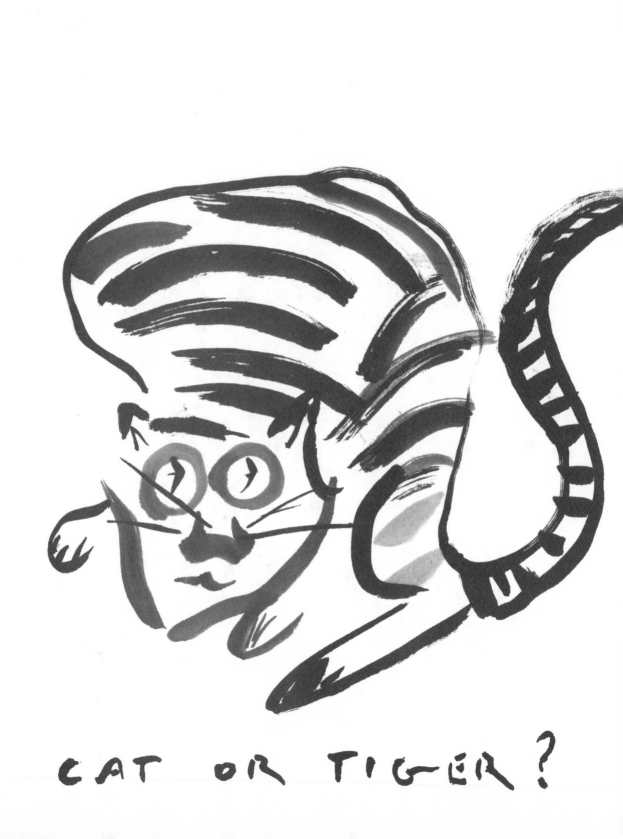

CAT OR TIGER?

Have you ever watched a cat waiting patiently to catch a mouse? Every cell is alert, all the way from the tip of his whiskers to the very end of his tail.

Whatever we do, whether walking, or standing, or cooking a meal, has the power to enliven us in the same way. When we bring our full attention to what we do, we naturally become more awake.

When you slice a peach or an apple, feel the texture of its skin through your fingertips. How gently or tightly do you hold it?

Notice the temperatures of what you touch; the coolness of lettuce when you first take it from the refrigerator, or the warmth of tomatoes that have been ripening in the sunshine.

Feel the weight and balance of the knife in your hand as you are slicing vegetables. How much or how little pressure is needed to cut a tomato, an onion, a zucchini, a carrot?

When you knead bread or cut vegetables, do you notice it's not just your hands that knead the dough or slice the onion? Feel how your arms, shoulders, legs—all of you—becomes involved.

Being there for the fullness of every action, no matter how common or small, wakes us up, "tuning us in" to a rich world of sensation and natural vitality.

Black Bean Chili

1 1/2 *cups dry black beans*

2 *tablespoons canola oil*

5 *medium garlic cloves, minced*

2 *medium yellow onions, chopped*

1 *tablespoon ground cumin*

1 *tablespoon dried oregano*

3 *tablespoons chili powder*

1 *teaspoon crushed red chili peppers*

2 *cups crushed tomatoes*

3 *jalapeño chili peppers, minced*

1 *cup chopped fresh pineapple or orange*
  (optional)

2 *tablespoons tamari*

Freshly ground pepper

Fresh cilantro, for garnish

SERVES 4 TO 6

Serve this chili topped with sour cream, chives, and grated cheese, or serve it with freshly made corn bread and a green salad.

If you don't have black beans on hand, use pinto or red kidney beans. The spices in the recipe are for a fairly hot chili, but you can adjust the amount of red chili peppers to your taste. Add fresh pineapple or orange for a zesty and surprising variation.

Sort through the beans for stones, which should be discarded. Rinse the beans and cover them with water in a large heavy pot. Bring to a full boil, drain, and rinse them again. Place in the pot with 6 cups of water. Bring to a simmer, cover with a lid, and cook for 2 hours.

When the beans have cooked for 1 hour, heat the oil in a large skillet. Sauté the garlic and onions over high heat for 3 to 4 minutes, stirring frequently. When the onions begin to look translucent, lower the heat to medium and stir in the cumin, oregano, chili powder, and crushed red chili pepper. Cook for 3 to 4 minutes, then add the tomatoes and jalapeños. Simmer for 10 minutes, stirring frequently.

Stir this chili sauce into the pot of beans. Add the pineapple or orange if using. Simmer partially covered for another hour until the beans are soft. Adjust the tastes to your liking. If you want more spice, add more jalapeños and crushed red pepper. As the chili simmers, keep the consistency as thick as a stew by adding more water if necessary.

Flavor with tamari and freshly ground pepper before serving. Garnish with fresh cilantro.

Variation: Chili Stew

Earthy and sweet vegetables are added to the basic chili recipe to make a thick, luscious stew. Serve over rice with sour cream and salsa on the side.

Follow the preceding chili recipe until the onions and garlic begin to look translucent. Add the carrots and turnips. Cook for a couple of minutes over high heat. Stir in the mushrooms and add the herbs and spices from the original recipe. Cook for 5 minutes, stirring frequently. If the vegetables begin to stick to the pan, stir in 1 tablespoon of water. Continue with the rest of the recipe. In this version, do not add the pineapple or orange.

1 cup ¼-inch-thick diagonally sliced carrots

1 cup finely chopped turnips

1 cup sliced mushrooms

Steamed Tortillas

In Mexico, every meal is served with a basket of hot freshly made tortillas. Heat the oven to 350 degrees and wrap a stack of tortillas in aluminum foil. Bake in the oven for 10 minutes. Serve wrapped in a cloth to keep the tortillas hot.

Refried Bean Burrito with Salsa Verde

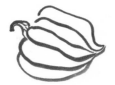

1 ½ cups dry pinto beans

4 tablespoons canola oil

7 medium-large garlic cloves, minced

2 tablespoons tamari

8 8-inch whole wheat tortillas

Salsa Verde (page 83)

2 cups red leaf lettuce, sliced in thin
    strips

Sour cream

1 ripe avocado

Lime juice and salt to taste

SERVES 4

Creamy and rich with garlic, these refried beans are delicious wrapped in tortillas and topped with Salsa Verde, sour cream, and avocado slices sprinkled with fresh lime juice.

Sort through the beans for stones, which should be discarded. Rinse the beans, place them in a large heavy pot, and cover with water. Bring to a full boil, drain, and rinse them again. Place in the pot with 6 cups of water. Bring to a simmer, cover with a lid, and cook for 2 hours, until soft.

When the beans have cooked, drain them, reserving the bean liquid. Heat the oil in a large skillet. Add the garlic and almost immediately, before the garlic begins to brown, stir in the beans. Cook them over medium-low heat, stirring with a wooden spoon. When the beans begin to thicken and cream together, add ½ cup of the reserved liquid. Continue cooking and when the beans seem dry, add another ½ cup of the bean liquid. Continue cooking in this way for 30 minutes, adding just enough liquid to keep the beans soft and creamy.

Preheat the oven to 350 degrees. Cover the tortillas with tinfoil and heat in the oven for 10 minutes.

Put about ⅓ cup of the refried beans in a strip down the center of each tortilla. Top with 2 or 3 tablespoons Salsa Verde and some lettuce. Roll the tortilla around the filling. Top with more salsa and a spoonful of sour cream. Cut the avocado into slices. Sprinkle with lime juice and salt to taste. Place the avocado slices on top of the tortilla. Garnish the plate with more thinly sliced lettuce and serve.

Bean Enchiladas

Enchiladas are tortillas that have been dipped in a sauce or salsa and baked around a filling. Fill these enchiladas with either Black Bean Chili or Refried Beans. For the sauce, use Ranchero Sauce or Red Pepper Sauce. Melt cheese on top if you wish, or serve garnished with sour cream, shredded lettuce, salsa, and fresh cilantro.

Preheat the oven to 350 degrees.

Spread half the sauce over the bottom of a 9 × 13-inch baking dish. Also spread a layer of sauce in the bottom of a shallow plate. Dip each tortilla in the plate to cover both sides with sauce. Place in the baking dish and fill the center of the tortilla with ⅓ cup of beans. Add 3 or 4 tablespoons of tomato salsa to the filling or some grated cheese if using. Roll the tortilla around the filling and place to the side in the baking dish. Repeat with all the tortillas. Cover the rolled tortillas with the rest of the sauce. Top with grated cheese and cover the baking dish with aluminum foil. Bake for half an hour.

Remove from the oven. Place 2 tortillas on each plate and scatter shredded lettuce on top. Garnish with tomato salsa, a dollop of sour cream, and cilantro.

3 to 4 cups Red Pepper Sauce (page 84) or Ranchero Sauce (page 183)

8 8-inch corn or whole wheat tortillas

3 cups refried beans (page 80) or Black Bean Chili (page 78)

2 cups Tomato Salsa (page 84)

2 cups grated Monterey Jack cheese (optional)

2 cups thinly sliced romaine or red leaf lettuce

Sour cream

Finely chopped fresh cilantro, for garnish

SERVES 4

Variation: Cheese Enchiladas

Instead of beans, fill the enchiladas with grated cheese, slices of avocado, olives, chopped fresh tomatoes, and Anaheim chili peppers. Bake with Salsa Verde for the sauce. Garnish with sour cream and cilantro.

Mushroom Enchiladas with Red Pepper Sauce

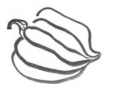

3/4 cup finely chopped Anaheim chili
   peppers

10 ounces firm tofu

1 tablespoon canola oil

1/2 medium yellow onion, finely chopped

3 medium garlic cloves, minced

3 cups sliced mushrooms

2 tablespoons canola oil

1 tablespoon tamari

1 teaspoon cumin powder

1 cup shredded Monterey Jack cheese

Salt

Cayenne

2 cups Red Pepper Sauce (page 84)

8 8-inch corn or whole wheat tortillas

Cilantro, for garnish

SERVES 4

These tasty enchiladas are filled with tofu ricotta, Anaheim chili peppers, and mushrooms. The spicy red pepper sauce has an elegant salmon color and is delicious with hints of cilantro and lime.

Remove the seeds and veins from the Anaheim chili peppers and set aside. Wash the tofu in cold water, drain in a colander, and set aside.

Heat the oil in a large pan. Sauté the onion and garlic over high heat for 3 to 4 minutes, stirring frequently. When the onions begin to look translucent, toss in the mushrooms and Anaheim chili peppers. Cook for a minute, add a tablespoon of water, and continue cooking for 5 to 10 minutes, until the mushrooms are well cooked.

In a large bowl, combine the tofu with the canola oil, tamari, and cumin, stirring until it looks like ricotta cheese. Stir the cooked mushrooms into the tofu, mix in the cheese, and season to taste with salt and cayenne.

Preheat the oven to 350 degrees. Spread a third of the sauce on the bottom of a 9 × 13-inch baking dish. Pour another third on a flat plate and dip each tortilla into the sauce, coating both sides. Place in the baking dish and spoon 1/3 cup of mushroom filling down the center of each tortilla. Roll the tortilla around the filling. Set to the side of the baking dish. Repeat with all 8 tortillas. If there is extra sauce left on the plate, cover the enchiladas with it. Cover the baking dish with aluminum foil and bake for 15 minutes, until hot.

Heat the remaining sauce on the stove. When the enchiladas come out of the oven, arrange them on a serving dish and pour the sauce over the top. Garnish with sprigs of cilantro and serve.

Salsa Verde

This "green" salsa is made with tomatillos, which look like small green tomatoes covered with a paperlike husk. They are lemon flavored, tart, and refreshing. This salsa is one of the best I have ever tasted. It is fast to make and will last for up to a week in the refrigerator.

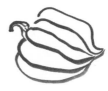

Peel and wash the tomatillos. In a medium pot, cover them with water and simmer for 5 to 10 minutes, until they are soft. Drain, saving the cooking liquid.

Wash the cilantro and pat dry. Cut the jalapeños in half and remove the seeds and veins. If fresh jalapeños aren't available, use the canned variety.

Place all the ingredients in a food processor and blend until smooth with ½ cup of the tomatillo cooking liquid. Chill in the refrigerator for 1 hour before serving.

1 pound tomatillos
2 cups tightly packed fresh cilantro
4 jalapeño chili peppers
¼ teaspoon salt

MAKES 2 CUPS

Tomato Salsa

4 serrano chili peppers

1 cup finely chopped plum tomatoes

3 tablespoons tomato paste

1/3 cup finely sliced scallions

2 large garlic cloves, minced

2 tablespoons chopped fresh cilantro

2 tablespoons fresh lime juice

1/2 cup water

Salt

Freshly ground pepper

MAKES 2 CUPS

While it may seem easier to buy already made salsa, nothing substitutes for the fresh tastes of lime, tomato, cilantro, and green onions. Serve this salsa with quesadillas or as a topping on bean enchiladas or tostadas.

Fresh serrano peppers are hot and vary in strength. Always taste as you go along to adjust for the spiciness of the salsa. This recipe is fairly hot.

Remove the veins and seeds of the peppers before mincing them. Combine all the ingredients, adding the serranos last, a tablespoon at a time. Taste to adjust the hotness.

Red Pepper Sauce

3 red peppers

Juice of 1/2 lime

1 tablespoon balsamic vinegar

3 medium garlic cloves, minced

1 plum tomato

2 tablespoons fresh cilantro

3 tablespoons canola oil

Pinch of cayenne

MAKES 2 CUPS

This spicy sauce, with its deep salmon color and mysterious hints of cilantro and lime, goes wonderfully with Mexican food. It's a quick sauce to make and good to have on hand for impromptu enchiladas or tostadas. It will keep for a week in the refrigerator.

Remove the seeds and veins of the peppers. Place all the sauce ingredients in a food processor and blend until smooth.

Tostadas

Tostadas make a quick lunch or light dinner. These crisp tortillas can be topped with all sorts of ingredients: fresh shredded lettuce, grated cheese, black olives, tomato salsa, refried beans, avocado slices, sour cream, or salsa verde. For parties, arrange bowls of these ingredients around a plate of tostadas and invite your guests to make their own.

Buy packaged corn tostadas in the markets or bake tortillas in the oven at 350 degrees, until crisp.

Tostadas with Red Pepper Sauce

Spread Red Pepper Sauce over the crisp tostadas. Cover with a layer of grated cheese and place under the broiler for a minute, until the cheese is melted. Top with sliced lettuce, tomato slices, and a dollop of sour cream. Sprinkle paprika on the sour cream and serve.

2 cups Red Pepper Sauce (page 84)

8 6-inch tostada shells

2 cups grated Monterey Jack cheese

2 cups thinly sliced red leaf lettuce

2 tomatoes, cut in half and sliced ¼ inch thick

Sour cream

Paprika for garnish

SERVES 4

Tostadas with Tomato Salsa, Avocado, and Black Olives

Spread a layer of salsa over the crisp tostadas. Cut the avocados in half, remove the pits, and peel off the skin. Cut into thin slices. Place the slices over the salsa. Scatter thinly sliced lettuce on top and garnish with 4 or 5 black olives.

2 cups Tomato Salsa (page 84)

8 6-inch tostada shells

2 ripe avocados

2 cups thinly sliced oak leaf lettuce

1 cup pitted and halved black olives

SERVES 4

Quesadillas

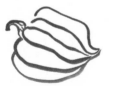

4 8-inch whole wheat tortillas

2 cups grated cheese: cheddar, Monterey
  Jack, or a mild chèvre

2 cups Tomato Salsa (page 84)

Sour cream

Chopped fresh cilantro, for garnish

SERVES 4

A quesadilla is the Mexican version of a grilled cheese sandwich. A tortilla is heated in a dry skillet, folded over grated cheese, and cooked until the cheese is melted. It is then topped with salsa, sour cream, and fresh chopped parsley or cilantro. Serve with guacamole on the side.

Whole wheat or corn tortillas are the tastiest. In addition to cheese, you can fill the quesadillas with chopped Anaheim or jalapeño chili peppers, tomato or avocado slices, chopped scallions, minced red onion, sautéed mushrooms, salsas, or chopped fresh cilantro.

Place a tortilla in a dry skillet over medium heat. Cover half the tortilla with grated cheese. Fold the other half over the cheese and press together with a spatula. Cook for 3 minutes, then flip the quesadilla over to its other side and cook 2 to 3 minutes, until the cheese is melted. Place on a plate in a warm oven until all are cooked.

Cut each quesadilla in wedges. Top with salsa, sour cream, and chopped cilantro for garnish.

Guacamole

There are many recipes for guacamole. Here is a simple version that tastes wonderful. For variety, add chopped tomatoes, a pinch of chili powder or cayenne, jalapeño peppers, minced scallions, or minced red onion.

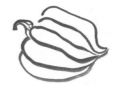

Cut the avocados in half and remove the pit. Scoop the avocado out of its shell into a medium mixing bowl. Mash it with a fork. Stir in the remaining ingredients. Season to taste with salt and freshly ground pepper. Always make guacamole just before serving.

2 ripe avocados

1 tablespoon fresh lemon juice

2 medium garlic cloves, minced

2 tablespoons chopped fresh cilantro

Salt

Freshly ground pepper

MAKES 2 CUPS

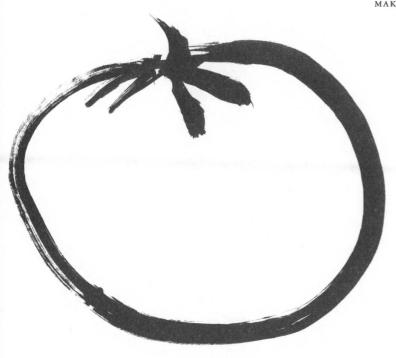

Jicama with Lime

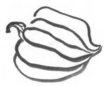

1 pound jicama

Juice of 1 lime

Pinch of cayenne

Watercress or cilantro, for garnish

SERVES 4

On the streets of Mexico vendors sell paper cones filled with sliced jicama sprinkled with cayenne pepper and a wedge of lime. It's a refreshing treat. Serve it on the side with quesadillas.

Peel the jicama and slice into julienne. Season to taste with the lime juice. Marinate for ½ hour in the refrigerator. Just before serving, season with cayenne and garnish with sprigs of watercress or cilantro.

Variation: Omit the cayenne and make a salad with julienned jicama, sliced oranges, and watercress drizzled with Chili Lime Basil Dressing (page 167).

These nachos were popular in our restaurant, The Beat'n Path Cafe. They are hearty enough for an entire meal, filling up the plate with a mound of beans, cheese, and toppings. If the chili is already made, they take no time to prepare.

Preheat the oven to 350 degrees. Place the tortillas flat on the oven rack and bake for 10 minutes, until crisp.

Place a crisp tortilla on a platter that can go under the broiler. Cover with a layer of warm chili. Scatter the top with grated cheese and place in the broiler for a minute or so, until the cheese has melted. Place on a serving plate, cut into quarters, and top with salsa, a dollop of sour cream, and scallions for garnish.

4 8-inch whole wheat tortillas

3 cups Black Bean Chili (page 78)

2 cups grated cheese (Monterey Jack or mild cheddar)

2 cups tomato salsa

Sour cream

1/2 cup finely sliced scallions, for garnish

SERVES 4

Sushi Ideas

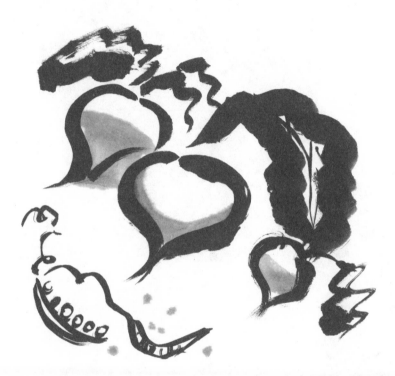

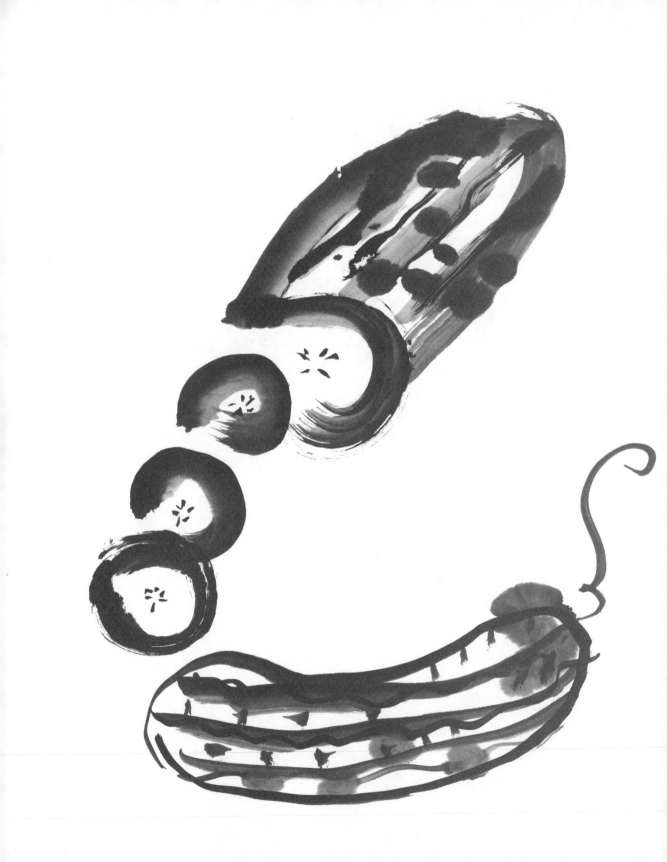

Every tradition speaks reverently of the breath. Our word spirit *comes from the Latin word for breath. The Greeks honored* pneuma, *the Indians* prajna, *the Chinese* chi, *and the Japanese* Ki. *All these words mean "breath."*

How well do you know your own breathing? What can you feel of it?

As your breath comes in and goes out, simply follow what happens in each inhalation, in each exhalation. Imagine that you are like an open window and feel how the air just comes in and goes out.

A simple awareness of breathing is used in many meditation disciplines, but you don't need to be somewhere peaceful and quiet to make this exploration. You can practice being aware of your breathing when you are shopping in the supermarket, or taking a walk, or cooking.

The kitchen can be your place of practice.

Be aware of your breathing when you are making a pie or stirring the soup. Notice what happens to it when you walk from place to place in the kitchen or when you reach into the cupboard to get a mixing bowl. You may discover that your breathing is responsive to everything you do.

What can you feel when you pick up a bag of heavy groceries?

You may notice that your breathing changes and so does your heartbeat. Other things change as well: Your muscles and tendons react. Your connection with the floor changes. Energy becomes available to you for the task.

It's enjoyable to be reminded of this life inside you and to feel how it constantly changes. As you become more intimate with your breathing, you may find yourself becoming more peaceful. You may notice other sensations, long forgotten or dulled, becoming clearer and clearer.

You can feel your breathing at any time: when you are standing in line for the bus, or when you are washing the dishes, or sitting at your desk. It's a touchstone that brings you closer to yourself in every moment.

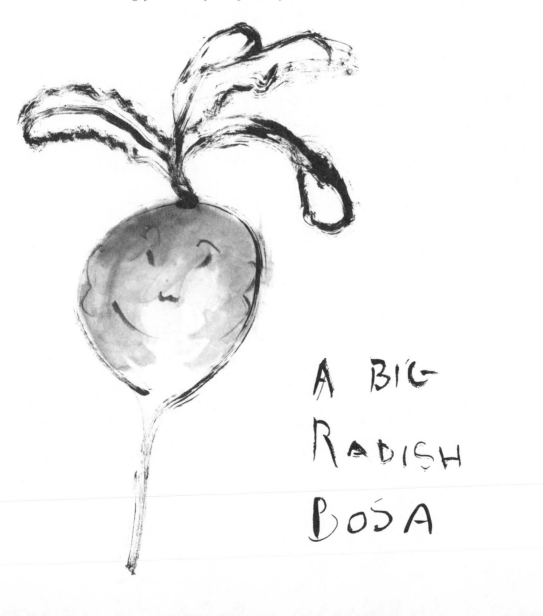

A BIG
RADISH
BOSA

Sushi

Sushi is always a treat and when you get the knack of it, it's very easy to make. The traditional ingredients for sushi, and the ones with which we are most familiar in sushi restaurants, are cucumber, pickled radish, tuna, crabmeat, and avocado. I have also included some recipes made with untraditional ingredients.

What You Need for Making Sushi

Bamboo Rolling Mat

Nori Seaweed: Square sheets of flat green-gold seaweed. Buy the variety that has been roasted. If it hasn't been roasted, briefly hold a sheet over the open flame of the stove until it turns a green-gold.

Wasabi: This very hot horseradish comes as a green powder. Sushi is traditionally served with a tiny mound of wasabi placed on the side of the plate. Mix the powder with water to a thick, doughy consistency and form it into a small square or triangular shape. Serve on the plate next to pickled ginger.

Gari (Sweet Pickled Ginger): These thin slices of pickled ginger are served in a small mound on the side of the plate and sometimes included in the filling.

Dipping Sauce: Serve a small bowl of dipping sauce with the sushi. The dipping sauce can be plain tamari, or tamari flavored with grated ginger, or combined with a small amount of wasabi powder. Wasabi is very hot, so add a little at a time to taste.

How to Roll Sushi

Place one sheet of toasted nori, shiny side down, on a bamboo rolling mat. With a dampened spoon, spread a ¼-inch-thick layer of sushi rice over the nori, leaving empty an inch at the bottom and 2 inches at the top. Starting 2 inches from the bottom, spread your filling ingredients in a 1-inch-wide strip over the rice from left to right.

Use the bamboo roller to fold the bottom of the nori over the filling. Roll away from you, pressing firmly with the roller. When you come to the end of the roll, press to shape the roll and remove the roller.

Wet a very sharp knife and cut the roll into 1-inch pieces. Place on a plate with the rice side showing. Serve with pickled ginger and a tiny mound of wasabi placed on the side of the plate.

Sushi Rice

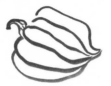

2 cups Japanese white rice

2 ½ cups water

⅓ cup mirin

3 tablespoons rice vinegar

½ teaspoon salt

MAKES 4 CUPS

The trick to making this rice is to cool it quickly while mixing in the mirin and vinegar. It's a good idea to enlist a friend for five or ten minutes to help fan the rice. Use a very good quality Japanese white rice.

Gently rinse the rice a couple of times until the water is clear. Drain it in a colander for half an hour. Place the rice and water in a heavy pot covered tightly with a lid. Cook over medium-high heat for 10 minutes until steam escapes the lid. Immediately turn the heat to low and cook for 10 to 15 minutes, until all the water has been absorbed. Remove from the heat and let the rice stand, covered, for 10 minutes.

In the meantime, heat the mirin, vinegar, and salt in a small saucepan until the salt is dissolved.

Put the cooked rice in a large mixing bowl. While vigorously fanning the rice to cool it, slowly stir in the mirin mixture. Continue stirring and fanning until the rice is cool. Use anything handy as a fan: A newspaper works well; I have sometimes even used a tiny hand-held electric fan.

Cucumber Sushi

Cucumber sushi is called Kappa Maki. For a variation to this recipe, include thinly grated carrots or avocado slices with the cucumbers.

Peel the cucumbers. Cut them lengthwise in half and scoop out the seeds with a spoon. Cut into strips about ¼ inch thick.

Place a sheet of toasted nori, shiny side down, on a bamboo rolling mat. With a dampened spoon, cover it with a thin layer of rice. Mix the powdered wasabi with 1 tablespoon of water to form a paste. Use your fingers to spread a thin line of wasabi across the rice from left to right. Place a ½-inch line of cucumber strips over the wasabi.

Using the bamboo roller, roll the sushi away from you. With a wet knife, cut the sushi into pieces 1 inch wide. Place a mound of wasabi and pickled ginger on the side of the plate and serve with a small dish of tamari to use as a dipping sauce.

2 medium-size cucumbers or 1 large cucumber
8 sheets toasted nori
4 cups Sushi Rice (page 96)
1 tablespoon wasabi powder
Pickled ginger
Tamari

SERVES 4
8 ROLLS 2 × 6 INCHES

Sweet Omelet Sushi

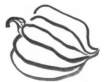

2 tablespoons mirin

2 eggs

1 tablespoon butter

8 sheets toasted nori

4 cups Sushi Rice (page 96)

1 tablespoon wasabi powder

Pickled ginger

Tamari

SERVES 4

8 ROLLS 2 × 6 INCHES

Make a few rolls of this sushi with just the omelet, and then vary it by including strips of sautéed mushrooms or spinach that has been lightly steamed. Sprinkle some toasted black sesame seeds over the rice. Garnish with pickled ginger and wasabi.

In a small bowl, whisk the mirin with the eggs. Heat the butter in a 12- or 14-inch skillet. Pour in the eggs and make a very thin omelet. Place on a plate to cool and cut into long thin strips.

Place a sheet of toasted nori, shiny side down, on a bamboo rolling mat. With a dampened spoon, cover the nori with a thin layer of rice. Mix the powdered wasabi with 1 tablespoon of water to form a paste. Use your fingers to spread a thin line of wasabi across the rice from left to right. Place a ½-inch line of omelet strips over the wasabi.

Using the bamboo roller, roll the sushi away from you. With a wet knife, cut the sushi into pieces 1 inch wide. Place a mound of wasabi and pickled ginger on the side of the plate and serve with a small dish of tamari to use as a dipping sauce.

California-Style Sushi

If using dried shiitake mushrooms, soak them in water for 30 minutes, until soft. Squeeze them dry. Remove the stems from the mushrooms and save them for soup stock. Slice the caps ¼ inch thick and sauté them in butter for 10 minutes. Add 1 tablespoon of water if they begin to stick to the pan. Toss with the lemon juice and remove from the heat.

Wash the green beans and trim the ends. Lightly steam until they are bright green and still crunchy. Cut the pepper in half, remove the seeds and veins, and slice into thin strips.

Place a sheet of toasted nori, shiny side down, on a bamboo rolling mat. With a dampened spoon, cover it with a thin layer of rice. Use your fingers to spread a thin line of wasabi across the rice from left to right. Place a strip of green beans over the wasabi. Place strips of the other ingredients on top, including the chopped pickled ginger.

Using the bamboo roller, roll the sushi away from you. With a wet knife, cut the sushi into pieces 1 inch wide. Place a mound of wasabi and pickled ginger on the side of the plate and serve with a small dish of tamari to use as a dipping sauce.

*4 ounces fresh or 2 ounces dried shiitake
   mushrooms*

1 tablespoon butter

1 teaspoon fresh lemon juice

12 green beans

1 poblano or Anaheim chili pepper

8 sheets toasted nori

4 cups Sushi Rice (page 96)

1 avocado, peeled and thinly sliced

½ cup chopped pickled ginger

Wasabi powder

Tamari

SERVES 4

8 SUSHI ROLLS 2 × 6 INCHES

Sushi Salad

2 cups Sushi Rice made with 2 cups rice
 (page 96)

2 ounces fresh or 1 ounce dried shiitake
 mushrooms

1 tablespoon butter

1 teaspoon lemon juice

2 cups snow peas

2 tablespoons black sesame seeds

1/2 large red pepper, sliced

1/4 cup chopped pickled ginger

1 sweet omelet (page 98), cut in strips

Tamari

SERVES 4

If you love the taste of the sweet vinegar rice used for sushi but don't have the time to make it into rolls, serve it as a rice salad tossed with your favorite sushi ingredients.

Prepare the rice and cool to room temperature.

If you use dried shiitakes, soak them for half an hour. When they are soft, squeeze them dry. Remove the stems from the mushrooms and save them for soup stock. Slice the caps and sauté them in the butter for 10 minutes. Add 1 tablespoon of water if they begin to stick to the pan. Drizzle with lemon juice and set aside.

Trim the ends of the snow peas. Lightly steam them for 2 to 3 minutes until they are bright green and still crunchy. Rinse under cold water and drain.

In a dry skillet, toast the sesame seeds over medium heat for 3 to 4 minutes, stirring frequently. When they smell fragrant, remove from the heat.

In a large serving dish, spread the red pepper slices, mushrooms, and snow peas with the sesame seeds and ginger over the rice and toss lightly. Cover the top with the omelet strips. Serve with tamari on the side in a small pouring bottle.

Vietnamese Spring Rolls

These spring rolls flavored with mint, basil, and chili are a Vietnamese version of sushi. They are traditionally served uncooked with a spicy peanut sauce or they can be deep-fried, resembling the well-known Chinese spring rolls.

Rice paper sheets are available in most Asian supermarkets. It took me a number of tries to learn how to use them. If you have never made these spring rolls before, try this recipe when you have time to experiment. Once you get the knack, it's easy.

1 10-ounce block firm tofu, cubed

1 tablespoon canola oil

10 mushrooms, sliced

1 tablespoon tamari

¼ cup Chili Lime Basil Dressing (page 167)

2 cups chopped mung bean sprouts

¼ cup chopped fresh mint

¼ cup chopped fresh basil

2 scallions, thinly sliced

½ red pepper, chopped

2 cups spinach, stems discarded, leaves cut into ½-inch strips

6 12-inch rice paper sheets

Asian-Style Peanut Sauce (page 165)

MAKES 6 LARGE ROLLS

Rinse the tofu in cold water and drain in a colander.

Heat the oil in a medium skillet. Sauté the mushrooms over medium-high heat for 5 minutes, stirring frequently. Toss in the tofu, add 1 tablespoon of water, and continue to cook for another 5 minutes, stirring with a spatula to prevent the tofu from sticking to the pan. Season with tamari, continue to cook another minute, and remove from the heat.

In a mixing bowl, toss the lime dressing with the bean sprouts, mint, basil, scallions, and the red pepper. Carefully wash and dry the spinach.

Fill a large bowl or pan with hot water. Quickly dip a sheet of rice paper into the water, then place it on a wet kitchen towel. Let it rest for 30 seconds until it becomes soft and pliable.

Starting 2 inches from the bottom, spread the mushrooms and tofu in a 2-inch-wide strip across the width of the rice paper, from left to right, leaving 2 inches on either side. Cover this with a strip of bean sprout mix and top with spinach.

Fold the 2-inch bottom of rice paper up over the filling. Fold the right and left sides toward the center, over the filling, like an envelope. Roll up and away from you, jelly-roll style. The rice paper will stick to itself, and should make a tight roll about 6 inches long and 2 inches wide.

Serve the roll as is, or cut it into thirds with a sharp wet knife. The filling has a tendency to fall out this way, so cut the roll only if it is very tight. Serve accompanied with small bowls of Asian-Style Peanut Sauce.

Variation: To fry the rolls, pour enough oil into a heavy skillet to reach a depth of 2 inches. Bring the oil to just below boiling. You can tell when the oil is ready by throwing a drop or two of water into it. If it sizzles, the oil is ready. Place 1 or 2 rolls in the oil and cook until crispy. Remove and drain on paper towels. Let the oil return to almost boiling before adding more rolls. Cut each roll into 3 pieces.

Pizzas and Vegetable Tarts

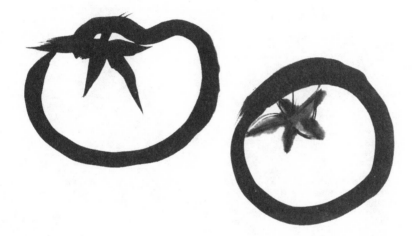

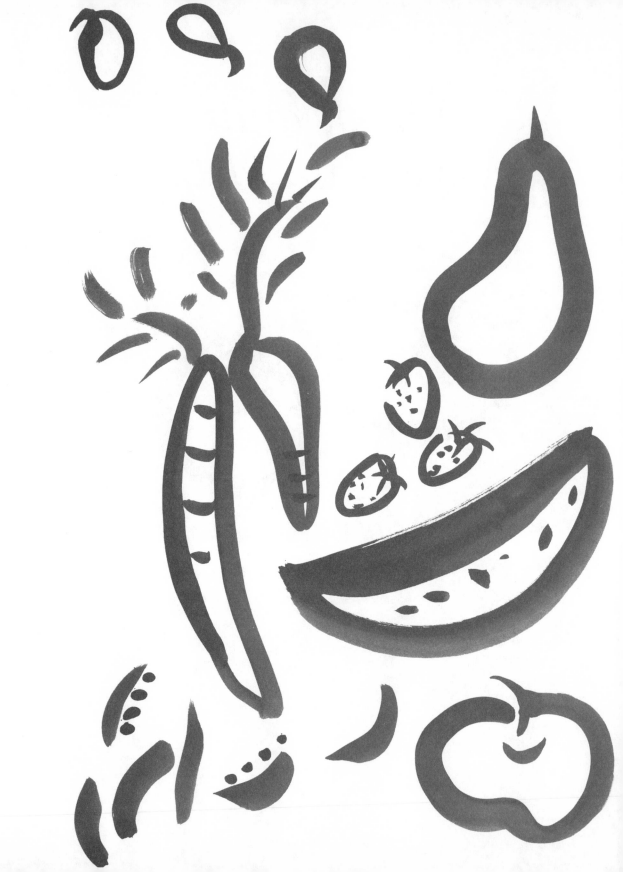

I used to teach cooking in a popular restaurant. When it got busy, my students would panic. It was always at this time that I offered my jewel of wisdom: "Cook with your feet."

This may sound like a strange recommendation, but it works.

Whatever you are doing right now, whether sitting in a chair or standing, could you become aware of what is under your feet and how you are in touch with it? Does it have strength—can it support you?

What can you feel of your feet and toes? Are they movable? Can they be in feeling touch with the ground?

The architecture of the foot is amazing. It's composed of twenty-six tiny bones connected to each other by as many joints, ligaments, tendons, and muscles, all movable in relation to one another.

As you are working in the kitchen, notice your connection with the floor. What does it feel like? Is is soft and springy? Is it hard?

Is there a place where you feel balanced in standing, where your weight evenly distributes through you?

The force of gravity on us is strong. Yet we can stand lightly on the ground.

Do you notice that it is not just your feet that meet the floor but your whole self? The top of your head, your shoulders, hip joints, and legs are all responsive to what is underneath you. Take time to feel this out as you walk, or sit, or stand.

As you experiment with this, you will begin to understand why martial artists have made awareness of gravity and the ground beneath them such an important part of their training. They call it being "rooted" and attribute their composure and strength to the living connection they arrive at with the earth.

Whole Wheat Pizza Dough

¹/₃ cup water

¹/₃ cup milk

¹/₂ teaspoon sugar

2 tablespoons active dry yeast

2 tablespoons olive oil

¹/₄ teaspoon salt

¹/₂ cup whole wheat flour

1 cup whole wheat pastry flour

ONE 12-INCH PIZZA

SERVES 4

Whole wheat flour gives pizza a nutty flavor, and while it's not as light as white flour, it's much more nourishing.

Preparing the dough is easy, but it does take time, so I generally double or triple the recipe and freeze the extra dough. To freeze, let it rise once, then punch it down. Wrap the dough tightly in plastic wrap, and place in the freezer. It will keep for up to four months. Before baking, let it warm up to room temperature, knead it for a minute, and then shape into a pizza.

In a small saucepan, heat the water, milk, and sugar to 110 to 115 degrees. It should be warm to the touch but not hot. Pour into a large mixing bowl and stir in the yeast. When the yeast has dissolved, mix in the olive oil and salt.

Sift the whole wheat flour and pastry flour together. Gradually stir the flour into the yeast and milk until the dough is soft enough to knead. It may still be a little sticky. Turn this out onto a lightly floured surface. Sprinkle flour on top and knead the dough for about 5 minutes, adding more flour as necessary.

Put the kneaded dough into a lightly oiled bowl. Cover with a cloth and let it rise for 30 minutes, until doubled in size.

Preheat the oven to 500 degrees.

Oil the pizza pan with olive oil. Place the dough on a lightly floured surface and roll it out to the size of the pizza pan. To make 4 single pizzas, cut the dough in quarters. Place on the pan and raise the edges of the dough slightly. Brush with olive oil and bake with your favorite toppings.

Mushroom Tomato Pizza

Smoked cheese goes perfectly with the earthy flavors of mushrooms and the sweet flavors of tomatoes. Use fresh shiitake mushrooms or wild mushrooms if they are available.

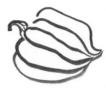

Prepare the pizza dough and let it rise.

Preheat the oven to 500 degrees.

Discard the stems from the shiitake mushrooms or save them for soup stock, and slice the caps. In a large skillet, heat the butter and oil and sauté all the mushrooms over high heat for 10 minutes, stirring frequently. They should be well cooked. Season to taste with salt and freshly ground pepper.

Roll out the dough and place it on a well-oiled pizza pan. Brush the dough lightly with olive oil and cover with a layer of cheese. Place the sautéed mushrooms over the pizza and arrange the sliced tomatoes on top. Brush the tomatoes with olive oil and scatter the garlic on top.

Bake for 10 to 15 minutes, until the crust is golden. Brush more olive oil on the edges of the crust and serve.

1 recipe Whole Wheat Pizza Dough (page 106)

1 cup thinly sliced fresh shiitake or other wild mushrooms (3 to 4 ounces)

1 tablespoon butter

1 tablespoon olive oil

2 cups sliced cultivated mushrooms

Salt

Freshly ground pepper

1 1/2 cups grated smoked mozzarella or smoked gouda cheese

2 plum tomatoes, thinly sliced

1 large garlic clove, minced

ONE 12-INCH PIZZA

SERVES 4

Summer Garden Pizza

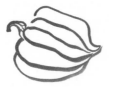

1 recipe Whole Wheat Pizza Dough
(page 106)

1 tablespoon olive oil

3 medium garlic cloves, minced

½ pound green beans, trimmed and
halved

1 tablespoon tamari

1 small red onion, sliced

⅓ cup finely chopped fresh basil

2 tablespoons fresh lovage or 1 sprig
fresh thyme

1 cup fresh corn kernels

1½ tomatoes, thinly sliced

Salt

Freshly ground pepper

¾ cup grated Parmesan cheese

Basil sprigs, for garnish

ONE 12-INCH PIZZA

SERVES 4

This is a particularly delicious pizza made with fresh vegetables from the garden that are lightly sautéed in garlic and olive oil, then baked with savory herbs.

Prepare the pizza dough and let it rise.

Preheat the oven to 500 degrees.

Heat the oil in a large sauté pan or wok. Add the garlic and, after a moment, toss in the green beans. Cook over medium-high heat for a couple of minutes, then add 2 or 3 tablespoons of water. Continue cooking for 5 minutes, stirring frequently, until the beans are half cooked. Season with tamari and remove from the heat.

Roll out the dough and place it on a well-oiled pizza pan. Brush it lightly with olive oil. Distribute the onions evenly over the dough. Place the green beans over the onions and scatter the fresh herbs and corn on top. Arrange the slices of tomato over the rest of the ingredients. Season with salt and freshly ground pepper, then scatter the top with grated Parmesan cheese.

Bake for 15 to 20 minutes, until the crust is golden. After baking, brush the edges with olive oil and garnish with sprigs of basil.

Here is another pizza that highlights tastes straight from the garden. Pesto is a summer sauce and it's wonderful on this pizza with lightly sautéed vegetables.

Prepare the pizza dough and let it rise.

Preheat the oven to 500 degrees.

Heat the oil in a sauté pan and lightly cook the squash over high heat for 5 minutes, stirring frequently, until al dente.

Roll out the dough and place it on a well-oiled pizza pan. Brush it lightly with olive oil and prebake for 10 minutes. Remove from the oven and cover with a layer of pesto (about 1 cup). Arrange the squash, tomatoes, and green pepper on top of the pesto. Return to the oven and bake for 5 minutes, until the crust is golden.

Remove the pizza from the oven. Brush the edges lightly with olive oil. Top with more pesto, ladling the sauce in swirls over the vegetables. The pesto may need thinning with water or a little oil. If so, taste for seasoning. Garnish with basil leaves and serve.

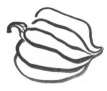

1 recipe Whole Wheat Pizza Dough (page 106)

1 tablespoon olive oil

2 to 3 yellow and green summer squash, sliced diagonally 1/4 inch thick

2 cups Pesto (page 164)

2 tomatoes, thinly sliced

1 green pepper, sliced in rounds

Fresh basil, for garnish

ONE 12-INCH PIZZA

SERVES 4

Pizza with Kale and Tofu

1 recipe Wheat Whole Pizza Dough
   (page 106)

½ pound kale

1 10-ounce block firm tofu

2 tablespoons olive oil

3 medium garlic cloves, minced

2 tablespoons lemon juice

1 tablespoon tamari

1 medium red onion, sliced thin

2 cups Basic Tomato Sauce (page 161)

½ cup grated Parmesan cheese

Finely chopped fresh parsley, for
   garnish

ONE 12-INCH PIZZA

SERVES 4

Kale is rich with minerals and vitamins and I love to cook with it. In this pizza, it is seasoned lightly with lemon and sautéed with tofu, which absorbs its sweet flavor.

Prepare the pizza dough and let it rise.

Preheat the oven to 500 degrees.

Remove the stems from the kale and coarsely chop the leaves. Rinse the tofu and drain in a colander. Cut in half, then into ⅓-inch-thick strips.

Heat the oil in a large wok or skillet. Add the garlic and cook for a moment over high heat. Before the garlic begins to brown, add the kale. Cook for 5 minutes, stirring frequently. Lower the heat to medium, add the tofu, and continue to cook for 10 or 15 minutes, until the kale is well cooked. Season with lemon juice and tamari.

Roll out the dough and place it in a well-oiled pizza pan. Brush the dough lightly with olive oil and prebake it for 10 minutes. Remove from the oven and evenly distribute the slices of onion over it. Cover with a layer of tomato sauce and arrange the kale and tofu on top. Pour the remaining tomato sauce in a circle. Return to the oven and bake another 10 minutes, until the crust becomes golden. Remove from the oven and brush the edges lightly with olive oil. Top with Parmesan cheese and garnish with parsley.

Potato and Red Pepper Pizza

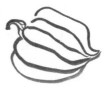

This is my favorite pizza and I love to surprise my friends with it. It never fails to delight them. Lovage is particularly wonderful with the potatoes, but if it isn't available use another herb such as sage or thyme.

Prepare the pizza dough and let it rise.

Preheat the oven to 500 degrees.

Heat the oil in a medium-size pan or wok. Add the garlic and onion and cook over high heat for 3 to 4 minutes, stirring frequently. Toss in the potatoes and herbs and cook for a minute. Turn the heat down to medium, add 2 tablespoons of water to prevent any sticking, and cover with a lid. Cook the potatoes for about 5 minutes, until half done. Uncover, add the red peppers, and cook for another 3 or 4 minutes, stirring frequently. Remove from the heat and season to taste with salt and freshly ground pepper.

Roll out the dough and place it in a well-oiled pizza pan. Brush the pizza dough lightly with olive oil. Cover with the potatoes and peppers. Arrange the olives on top and dust lightly with Parmesan cheese. Bake for 15 minutes, or until you are sure the potatoes are soft and the pizza is golden around the edges. Remove from the oven and brush the edges of the pizza with olive oil. Garnish with fresh parsley.

*1 recipe Whole Wheat Pizza Dough
(page 106)*

2 tablespoons olive oil

3 small garlic cloves, minced

1 cup thinly sliced red onion

*8 ounces new red potatoes, thinly sliced
(about 2 cups)*

*1 tablespoon chopped fresh lovage, sage,
or thyme*

1 large red pepper, cut in thin strips

Salt

Freshly ground pepper

*¾ cup Niçoise olives, pitted and cut in
half*

½ cup grated Parmesan cheese

*Finely chopped fresh parsley, for
garnish.*

ONE 12-INCH PIZZA

SERVES 4

Carrot and Beet Pizza

Believe it or not, this is a great pizza to make. The ingredients are simple, yet it turns out tasting rich and satisfying. The color of the sauce is a deep purple, and it looks elegant topped with steamed whole baby carrots and lightly sautéed beet greens.

1 recipe *Whole Wheat Pizza Dough* (page 106)

3 medium-size beets with fresh leafy green tops (about 1¾ pounds)

2 tablespoons canola oil

3 garlic cloves, minced

1 medium yellow onion, chopped

4 medium carrots, cut into ½-inch slices

1½ cups water

6 or 7 tiny whole baby carrots, for topping

1 tablespoon canola oil

Salt

Freshly ground pepper

2 tablespoons tamari

1 teaspoon balsamic vinegar

ONE 12-INCH PIZZA

SERVES 4

Prepare the pizza dough and let it rise.

Cut off the beet leaves, leaving a little of the stem. Wash the beets and greens. Slice the greens ¼ inch thick (you should have about 2 cups) and set aside.

Peel the beets and cut them into ½-inch slices. Heat the canola oil in a large sauté pan. Add the garlic and onion, and cook over high heat for 3 to 4 minutes, stirring frequently. When the onion begins to look translucent, stir in the beets and carrots. Continue to cook over high heat for 5 minutes. Add the water, cover the pan with a lid, lower the heat, and simmer for 20 minutes, until the vegetables are soft.

In the meantime, steam the whole baby carrots. Drain and set aside.

In a small skillet, heat the oil and sauté the beet greens and stems over high heat for 2 minutes, stirring frequently. Season to taste with salt and freshly ground pepper. Set aside.

Preheat the oven to 500 degrees.

In a food processor, blend the cooked beets and carrots until smooth. Add the tamari and balsamic vinegar. Season to taste with salt and freshly ground pepper.

Roll out the dough and place it in a well-oiled pizza pan. Brush the pizza dough with olive oil and prebake it for 10 minutes. Cover with a layer of beet and carrot sauce. Arrange the whole baby carrots on top, brush them with olive oil, and return to the oven and bake for 5 to 10 minutes, until the crust is golden.

Brush the edges of the pizza with olive oil. Arrange the beet greens on top and serve.

Bruschetta with Tomatoes and Basil

Bruschetta is an Italian midday snack made with slices of thick crusty bread toasted over a fire and drizzled with olive oil and garlic. To make it even more irresistible, we add tomatoes and fresh basil. The key to this recipe is the bread. The best bruschetta is made with fresh thick-crusted country bread.

In a medium bowl, mash the garlic and salt together with the back of a spoon or a pestle. Stir in the olive oil, tomatoes, and basil.

Cut the bread into slices ½ inch thick. Toast them in the broiler or on top of a grill. Spoon the olive oil and tomatoes mixture over the bread and serve. Bruschetta goes well with soup and a simple salad, or serve it with roasted vegetables.

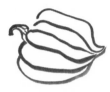

2 medium garlic cloves, minced

Pinch of salt

¼ cup olive oil

¾ cup chopped plum tomatoes

⅓ cup finely chopped fresh basil

4 thick slices of Italian, French, or sourdough bread

SERVES 4

Vegetable Tarts

These tarts are made with a custard of tofu cream. They are easy to make and much lighter than traditional tarts filled with heavy cream and cheese. Experiment with your own combinations of vegetables; the tofu cream stays the same. Make a tart with artichoke hearts or tomatoes and spinach. I once made an exotic one for Thanksgiving with cranberries and winter squash.

Whole Wheat Tart Pastry

1 cup whole wheat pastry flour

¼ teaspoon salt

6 tablespoons butter

¼ cup cold water

ONE 9-INCH TART

The secret to making this crust is to handle the dough as little as possible. Roll it out on a marble or tile surface only five or six times. Don't go over and over it. Once in the pie plate, scallop the edges using your left thumb, pinching the dough around it with your right thumb and forefinger.

In a large bowl, sift the flour and salt together. Cut the butter into small pieces and then crumble it into the flour using your fingers. Pour in the water a little at a time, mixing lightly with a spoon or fork, until the dough comes together into a ball. Refrigerate for half an hour.

Sprinkle a marble or tile surface with flour. Form the dough into a flat circle and sprinkle some flour on top and on your rolling pin. Roll away from you 5 or 6 times until it is the size of the pie plate. Keep moving the dough to make sure it doesn't stick to the marble surface. Fold in half, pick it up, and unfold in the pie plate. Use a small knife to trim the edges, then scallop them with your fingers.

Pepper Tart

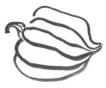

If you love peppers, this is for you. Their red, yellow, and orange colors are a delight for the eye in this tart served with black olives.

Preheat the oven to 350 degrees.

To make the tofu cream, wash the tofu and drain in a colander for a couple of minutes. In a food processor, blend the tofu, eggs, oil, tamari, and mustard until smooth.

Wash the peppers, cut them in half, and remove the veins and seeds. Slice them lengthwise and in half, so that each piece is bite-size and thin.

Heat the oil in a large skillet. Sauté the garlic and onion over high heat for 3 to 4 minutes, stirring frequently. When the onions begin to look translucent, add the peppers and continue to cook for 10 minutes.

Mix the cooked peppers in a large bowl with the tofu cream, basil, and olives. Season to taste with salt and freshly ground pepper. Pour into the tart shell, smoothing the top, and cover with Parmesan cheese. Bake in the oven for 45 minutes, or until the surface is golden and the custard has set. Before serving, let it cool for 10 minutes.

1 recipe Whole Wheat Tart Pastry
  (page 114)

FOR THE TOFU CREAM:
1 10-ounce block firm tofu

2 eggs

2 tablespoons canola oil

2 tablespoons tamari

2 teaspoons Dijon mustard

2 medium red peppers

2 medium yellow or orange peppers

1 tablespoon olive oil

2 medium garlic cloves, minced

1 medium red onion, chopped

1 cup chopped fresh basil

1 cup halved and pitted black Niçoise
  olives

Salt

Freshly ground pepper

¼ to ½ cup grated Parmesan cheese

ONE 9-INCH PIE

Swiss Chard and Tomato Tart

FOR THE TOFU CREAM:

1 10-ounce block firm tofu

2 eggs

2 tablespoons canola oil

2 tablespoons tamari

1 tablespoon olive oil

1 medium yellow onion, chopped

2 large garlic cloves, minced

1 teaspoon turmeric

*8 to 10 cups coarsely chopped Swiss
    chard (about ¾ pound)*

½ cup chopped parsley

2 tomatoes

Salt

Freshly ground pepper

*1 recipe Whole Wheat Tart Pastry
    (page 114)*

¼ to ½ cup grated Parmesan cheese

ONE 9-INCH TART

This creamy tart is flavored with the mild sweetness of Swiss chard and tomatoes. It is a beautiful golden color with specks of green and red.

Preheat the oven to 350 degrees.

To prepare the tofu cream, rinse the tofu in cold water and drain it in a colander for a couple of minutes. Place the tofu, eggs, oil, and tamari in a food processor and blend until smooth.

Heat the oil in a large pot. Sauté the onion and garlic over high heat for 3 to 4 minutes, stirring frequently. When the onions begin to look translucent, stir in the turmeric and cook for another minute. Mix in the Swiss chard. Lower the heat to medium and cook for 10 minutes, until the chard has cooked down. Remove from the heat and set aside.

In a large bowl, mix the tofu cream with the chard and parsley. Slice the tomatoes in half and then in thin slices. Gently stir in half of them and set the other half aside. Season to taste with salt and freshly ground pepper. Pour into the pie shell. Arrange the rest of the tomatoes on top and cover with Parmesan cheese. Bake for 45 minutes, or until the custard has set and is golden. Cool for 10 minutes before serving.

Vegetable Dishes

THIS MATTER

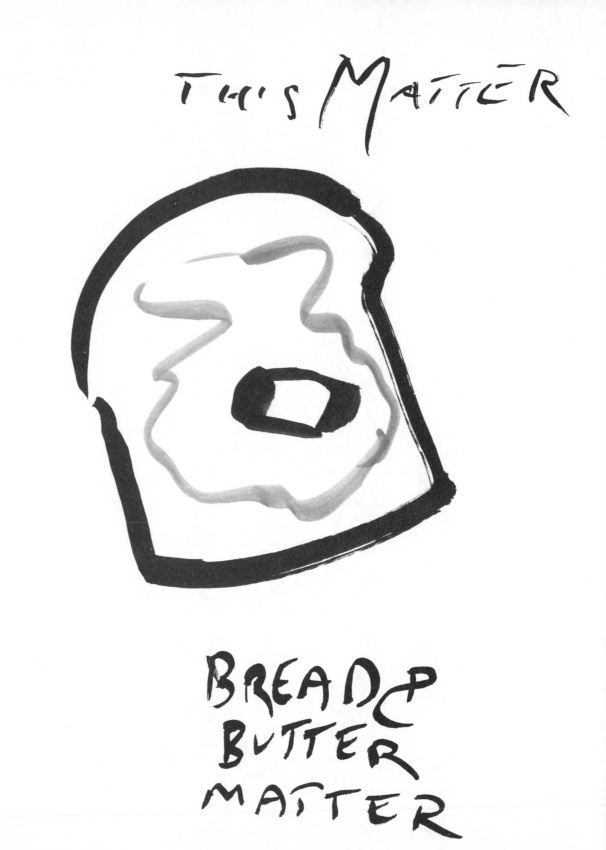

BREAD&
BUTTER
MATTER

When I practice the Tea Ceremony I am often reminded of the Tea master Rikyu's suggestion that heavy utensils, such as the iron kettle filled with water, be lifted so as to appear almost weightless and that light objects, like the small bamboo tea scoop, be held as though possessing a mysterious weight.

In the kitchen you can bring this presence to all your actions just by being more attentive.

As you wash the dishes, notice how your fingers curl around the edges of a plate or cup, feeling its shape and size. Become aware of the texture of smooth porcelain or the roughness of pottery. Feel the weight of each dish.

When you have thoroughly explored one dish, pick up another and explore it with this same sense of newness. Feel the sensations that come from the object in your hands; the perfect roundness of a bowl, the delicate weight of a wineglass, the delightful balance of a fork or spoon, each time realizing more fully the potential of your sense of touch.

As you try this out, you may become aware of your breathing. Notice too how you are standing. Perhaps you can feel how the weight of each object influences you.

What happens when you reach to the top shelf to put a bowl away? Your arms may need to find a different way of holding it for more balance. Become aware of your connection with the floor. Does it support you as you reach to put away the dishes?

Take time to feel what is most natural and easy.

The Zen master Suzuki Roshi said that there is no such thing as an enlightened person, there is just enlightened activity. By arriving at an attitude of quiet curiosity, even the most common task becomes an opportunity to explore our nature.

Vegetable Dishes

Early one summer I stopped at a roadside vegetable stand whose sign advertised KILLER CORN. The corn was just picked that morning and the farmer was enthusiastic about it. He offered us a freshly shucked ear of corn with a bit of lime juice squeezed over it. It was unbelievably delicious!

This experience reminded me of some of the simple ways to enjoy vegetables that sometimes, in our haste for the new, we forget to cook for our friends and family.

Many of the dishes that follow can be served alongside a simple rice pilaf and a salad to make a delicious light meal, but most of them can be the main course offerings. Hot and Spicy Cajun Shish Kebabs are great with roasted corn on the cob and coleslaw. Southwestern Potato Pancakes can be served with Cilantro Pesto and broiled tomatoes. Roasted Autumn Vegetables served with a garlicky bruschetta is sometimes all that is needed for a satisfying and delightful meal.

Baked Tomatoes

Tomatoes baked in the oven become richly sweet and juicy. This is a great dish to serve with wild rice pilaf or grilled polenta.

Preheat the oven to 350 degrees.

Mix the bread crumbs, Parmesan, and herbs together in a food processor.

Place the tomatoes face up in a broiling pan. Cover the tops with the bread crumb mixture. Bake for 45 minutes and serve garnished with fresh basil leaves.

Variation: Broiled Tomatoes with Cilantro Pesto

Preheat the broiler. Cut the tomatoes in half. Place face up in a broiling dish. Layer the tops with Cilantro Pesto (page 164) and cover with plain fine bread crumbs. Place in the lowest rack of the broiler and cook until the tops are browned.

½ cup fine bread crumbs

¼ cup grated Parmesan cheese

2 tablespoons finely chopped fresh basil

½ teaspoon finely chopped fresh marjoram

4 large ripe tomatoes, cut in half

Fresh basil leaves, for garnish

SERVES 4

Baked New Potatoes with Rosemary

Cut small red potatoes in halves or quarters and toss them with finely chopped fresh rosemary, salt, freshly ground pepper, and just enough olive oil to coat them lightly.

Bake for 1 hour in the oven at 350 degrees. Toss every so often to brown them on all sides. Serve plain or with sour cream. They go wonderfully with a green salad and steamed vegetables.

Roasted Japanese Eggplants with Sesame Butter

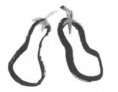

Trim and slice the small eggplants lengthwise. Place them in a colander, sprinkle with salt, and let them sit for half an hour. Rinse well and pat dry. Lay them face up in a shallow broiling dish. Brush well with olive oil and broil for 5 to 10 minutes. Top with Spicy Sesame Butter and garnish with chopped fresh cilantro.

6 Japanese eggplants

½ teaspoon salt

Olive oil

1 cup Spicy Sesame Butter (page 169)

Fresh cilantro, finely chopped for
*   garnish*

SERVES 4

VEGETABLE DISHES

Cauliflower Gratin

My mother showed me how to make this dish. It is one of my favorites, and very easy to make.

Preheat the oven to 350 degrees.

Leave the cauliflower whole, or separate it into large florets and steam until half cooked, about 6 to 8 minutes. Place it in a 2-quart casserole and pour the béchamel sauce over it.

Combine the bread crumbs and Parmesan. Cover the cauliflower with the bread crumb mixture. Bake, covered with aluminum foil, for 20 minutes. Uncover and continue to bake another 10 minutes, until the top is browned and the cauliflower is soft. Garnish with parsley or fresh basil leaves.

Variation: To give the cauliflower more color and flavor, add sliced tomatoes to the top before covering with the Parmesan and bread crumbs. When the tomatoes bake, their juices merge with the cauliflower.

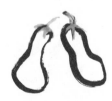

1 2½-pound head cauliflower, leaves trimmed

2 cups Béchamel Sauce (page 163)

1 cup fine bread crumbs

½ cup grated Parmesan cheese

Finely chopped fresh parsley or basil leaves, for garnish

SERVES 4

Zucchini Fritters

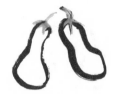

1 tablespoon olive oil

3 large garlic cloves, minced

1 cup chopped red onion

1 teaspoon chopped fresh thyme

1 tablespoon chopped fresh basil

4½ cups grated zucchini (about 4
   medium zucchini)

Salt

Freshly ground pepper

¼ cup chopped fresh parsley

20 black olives, chopped

½ cup whole wheat pastry flour

3 tablespoons grated Parmesan cheese

4 eggs, separated

Butter or canola oil for frying

MAKES 8 LARGE FRITTERS

SERVES 4

These zucchini fritters are delicious served with a tomato sauce, a béchamel sauce, or topped with sweet red pepper relish. They can be served warm or cool. Like most pancakes, you need to have a good skillet. If you have two pans cooking at the same time, these fritters will be done in no time at all.

Heat the olive oil in a large skillet. Sauté the garlic and onion over high heat for 3 to 4 minutes, stirring frequently. When the onions begin to look translucent, stir in the herbs. Cook for 1 minute, then add the zucchini. Reduce the heat to medium and cook for 5 minutes. Remove from the heat and season to taste with salt and freshly ground pepper. Stir in the chopped parsley and the olives. Set aside.

In a separate bowl, mix the flour and Parmesan together. Stir into the zucchini mixture. Whisk the egg yolks in a small bowl and add them to the zucchini. Beat the egg whites until stiff and fold into the batter.

Heat a skillet or griddle over medium heat and butter or oil it lightly. When it starts to sizzle, ladle a large spoonful of zucchini batter onto the griddle and cook until lightly browned. Turn and cook on the other side for a minute or two until brown. Repeat, using all the batter. Make sure you keep your griddle well oiled. These fritters are good served hot or at room temperature.

Potato Provençal

This casserole dish is rich with a variety of Mediterranean flavors.

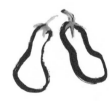

Cook the potatoes by steaming them for 5 minutes or until they are half cooked and still firm. Drain and set aside.

Preheat the oven to 350 degrees.

Heat the oil in a small skillet. Sauté the garlic, onions, and herbs over high heat for 3 to 4 minutes, stirring frequently. When the onions become translucent, remove from the heat. In a medium bowl, carefully mix the cooked potatoes with the onions. Season with tamari and freshly ground pepper.

Assemble all the ingredients in a 2-quart casserole: Place half the potatoes and onions in the bottom of the dish, cover with half the tomatoes and olives, and top with ½ cup of Parmesan cheese. Continue layering in this order until all the ingredients are used.

Bake in the oven, covered loosely with foil, for 30 minutes. Uncover and continue to bake for 20 minutes, until brown on top. Garnish with parsley.

1 pound new red potatoes, sliced ⅓ inch thick

3 tablespoons olive oil

4 garlic cloves, minced

2 medium red onions, sliced thin

1 tablespoon crushed fresh lovage, or fresh sage

1 tablespoon chopped fresh thyme

1 teaspoon tamari

Freshly ground pepper

4 tomatoes, thinly sliced in half (about ¾ pound)

1 cup pitted and halved black olives

1 cup grated Parmesan cheese

Finely chopped fresh parsley, for garnish

SERVES 4

Butternut, Sweet Potatoes, Carrots, and Ginger

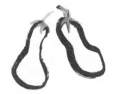

1 pound butternut squash

4 medium carrots, sliced

2 pounds sweet potatoes, peeled and
 sliced

3 inches fresh ginger

3 tablespoons butter

2 tablespoons tamari

Salt

Freshly ground pepper

SERVES 4 TO 6

This is a great dish for Thanksgiving as well as every day. It is sweet, delicious, and easy to make.

Peel the butternut squash and scoop out the seeds. Cut all the vegetables the same size, about ⅓ inch thick. Place them in a steamer and cook until soft, about 20 minutes.

Peel and finely grate the ginger. Place all the ingredients in a food processor and blend until smooth. Season to taste with salt and freshly ground pepper. Place in a baking dish and keep warm in the oven until serving.

Hot and Spicy Cajun Shish Kebabs

Cayenne and lots of paprika spice up these shish kebabs. They are delicious served on a bed of rice mixed with a little Parsley Pesto (page 164) or served alongside grilled polenta.

Preheat the broiler or start a charcoal fire.

Mix together the dry spices and herbs.

In a medium mixing bowl, combine the olive oil, lemon juice, and garlic. Stir in the dry spice mix and cayenne.

Thread the vegetables onto a bamboo skewer. Brush them thickly with the Cajun sauce, turning so that all sides are well coated.

If broiling in the oven, place the shish kebabs in a baking dish, brush more sauce on top, and broil for about 5 minutes, turning frequently. If grilling on a barbecue, place the shish kebabs over medium-hot coals. Grill 5 to 7 minutes on each side.

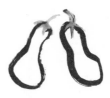

2 tablespoons paprika

2 teaspoons salt

2 teaspoons ground black pepper

1 teaspoon dried oregano

1 teaspoon dried thyme

1 bay leaf, crushed

1/4 teaspoon dried orange or lemon peel

1/4 cup olive oil

2 tablespoons lemon juice

1 garlic clove, minced

1/8 to 1/4 teaspoon cayenne

2 to 3 yellow squash and zucchini, cut into 1/2-inch-thick rounds

1 pound cherry tomatoes

10 cultivated mushrooms

2 red peppers, 2 green peppers, and 2 yellow or orange peppers, cut into squares

SERVES 4 TO 6

Roasted Autumn Vegetables

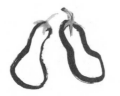

3 new red potatoes, cut into bite-size
    pieces

1 sweet potato, cut into bite-size pieces

1 red pepper, sliced in thin strips

1 green pepper, sliced in thin strips

1 red onion, sliced

1 1-pound acorn squash, cut in half
    and sliced 1/4 inch thick

1/2 pound green beans, ends trimmed

2 medium zucchini, cut diagonally 1/2
    inch thick

Extra virgin olive oil

Fresh minced rosemary

Salt

Freshly ground pepper

SERVES 4

Roasting is one of the best ways to feature autumn vegetables. It's a simple way of cooking. The olive oil and salt concentrate the flavors of these vegetables so they become sweeter and more intense. When serving, arrange them on a large platter, varying shape and color.

Preheat the oven to 500 degrees.

Using one large mixing bowl, toss each group of vegetables separately with olive oil, 1 teaspoon fresh rosemary, salt, and freshly ground pepper. Use just enough oil to lightly coat the vegetables. Spread the vegetables in a single layer in a large baking dish or pan. Keep the different vegetables separate. Some will take longer to roast than others. The potatoes and acorn squash take about 40 minutes, the zucchini and green beans about 15 minutes, and the peppers and onion roast for 10 minutes.

During roasting, turn the vegetables every so often so they brown on all sides. Remove from the oven as they become tender and arrange on a serving plate. Cool to room temperature and serve.

Southwestern Potato Pancakes

These flavorful potato pancakes are made with corn and green chilis. Top with Cilantro Pesto or sour cream. Masa harina is a fine cornmeal easy to find in Spanish markets or supermarkets.

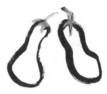

Preheat the oven to 350 degrees.

Wash the potatoes, prick them all over with a fork, and bake in the oven for 40 minutes, until soft in the center. Cut the Anaheim chilis in half lengthwise, discard the veins and seeds, and coarsely chop them.

In a large bowl, mix the masa harina with the baking powder. Cut the baked potatoes in half and scoop the potato into the bowl. Add the chilis, corn kernels, cheese, salsa, and seasonings. Slowly stir in enough water for the mixture to hold together to form into patties.

Heat the butter and oil in a large skillet and fry the patties on both sides until brown and crispy. Serve topped with Cilantro Pesto or sour cream.

1 pound baking potatoes

2 Anaheim chili peppers or ½ cup chopped canned green chilis

2 cups masa harina

1 teaspoon baking powder

1 cup corn kernels

1 cup grated cheddar cheese

1 to 2 tablespoons tomato salsa

Salt

Freshly ground pepper to taste

1 tablespoon butter and 1 tablespoon canola oil for frying

Cilantro Pesto (page 164) or sour cream

SERVES 4 TO 6

Stuffed Zucchini

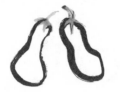

6 *medium zucchini*

2 *tablespoons olive oil*

2 *garlic cloves, minced*

1 *cup chopped mushrooms*

1 *teaspoon minced fresh marjoram or ½ teaspoon dried marjoram*

¼ *teaspoon ground cloves*

¼ *teaspoon grated nutmeg*

⅓ *cup white wine*

1 *cup fine bread crumbs*

½ *cup grated Parmesan cheese*

1 *tablespoon tamari*

Freshly ground pepper

SERVES 4

This dish is quick to make and always looks elegant.

In a large pot, steam the zucchini whole for 5 minutes until tender but still firm. Remove from the steamer and drain. Trim the ends and cut in half lengthwise. Scoop out the center, making enough of a hollow for the stuffing.

Heat the oil in a medium skillet. Sauté the garlic and the mushrooms over high heat, stirring frequently. After a couple of minutes add the marjoram, cloves, and nutmeg. When the mushrooms are almost done, about 8 minutes, pour in the white wine and continue to cook for 5 minutes over high heat until reduced. Remove from the heat and set aside.

In a separate bowl, combine the bread crumbs, ¼ cup Parmesan cheese, and the cooked mushrooms. Season with tamari and freshly ground pepper.

Preheat the oven to 350 degrees. Oil a baking dish large enough to contain all the zucchini placed in one layer. Fill the centers of the zucchini with the stuffing. Top with the rest of the Parmesan and bake for 30 minutes, until brown.

Ratatouille

Although there are many good recipes for ratatouille, it is such a versatile and delicious dish, I must include a version for this book. Serve it with polenta or steamed rice; it is an excellent filling for crepes, roulades, and quiche. It's also a good topping for pizza.

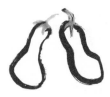

Heat the oil in a large heavy pot. Add the garlic and onion and cook over medium heat, stirring frequently. After a minute, stir in the thyme, rosemary, and basil. Continue cooking for 3 or 4 minutes, until the onions look translucent. Toss in the eggplant. Reduce the heat to medium and cook for 10 minutes. Add the zucchini and continue cooking another couple of minutes. Stir in the tomatoes, tomato paste, and ½ cup water. Cover with a lid, reduce the heat to low, and simmer for 30 minutes.

Add the red wine. Continue cooking another 10 minutes. Stir in the green peppers and tamari. Season to taste with freshly ground pepper. Remove from the heat when the peppers turn bright green and are tender yet still crunchy, about 5 minutes. Garnish with parsley and serve accompanied with Parmesan cheese.

2 tablespoons olive oil

4 garlic cloves, minced

1 small yellow onion, chopped

¾ teaspoon dried thyme

½ teaspoon dried rosemary

2 tablespoons dried basil

4 cups peeled and cubed eggplant (1-pound eggplant)

3 medium zucchini, cut in bite-size pieces (about ¾ pound)

2 cups coarsely chopped fresh tomatoes

2 tablespoons tomato paste

¼ cup red wine

2 medium green peppers, cut into thin strips

1 tablespoon tamari

Freshly ground pepper

Finely chopped fresh parsley for garnish

Grated Parmesan cheese to serve on the side

SERVES 4

Spicy Aduki Beans

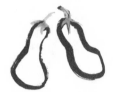

½ cup dry aduki beans

4 cups water

1 tablespoon canola oil

1 medium yellow onion, chopped

5 garlic cloves, minced

3 medium sweet potatoes, peeled and cut
    into bite-size pieces (1 ½ cups)

1 cup bite-size pieces carrots

4 inches ginger, peeled and grated

2 tablespoons tamari

Cayenne

SERVES 4

Aduki beans are delicious simmered with ginger, carrots, and sweet potatoes. Use lots of ginger, the spicier the better! Serve with rice, topped with sour cream for elegance.

Sort through the beans for stones, which should be discarded. Rinse the beans and place them in a large pot with the water, partially cover with a lid, and bring to a simmer.

Heat the oil in a large wok or sauté pan. Add the onion and garlic and cook over high heart for 3 to 4 minutes. Stir in the sweet potatoes and carrots. Continue to cook over high heat for 5 minutes, stirring frequently. Remove from the heat and add to the pot of beans. Stir in the ginger, cover with the lid, and continue to simmer for 1 hour, until the beans, carrots, and potatoes are soft.

After half and hour, taste to see if there is enough ginger. It should be very spicy. The strength of ginger varies depending on its freshness. Add more if needed. Season with tamari and cayenne.

Stir-Fry Tofu

This is one of my favorite ways to cook tofu, and I generally make a lot of it at one time. It keeps well in the refrigerator and I use it in salads and eat it plain (some people think it tastes like chicken). Serve it topped with Cilantro Pesto (page 164) or dip it in sweet and hot Thai sauces.

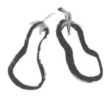

Wash the tofu in cold water and drain it in a colander for ½ hour. Cut it into ¼- or ½-inch-thick cubes.

Heat the oil and butter in a large skillet. Toss in the tofu and cook over high heat continuously turning the tofu to brown it on all sides.

Stir in the tamari and continue to cook for 2 to 3 minutes. The tamari will sear into the tofu and flavor it. Remove from the heat and cool for 5 minutes before serving.

1 10-ounce block firm tofu

1 tablespoon canola oil

1 tablespoon butter

2 tablespoons tamari

Salads

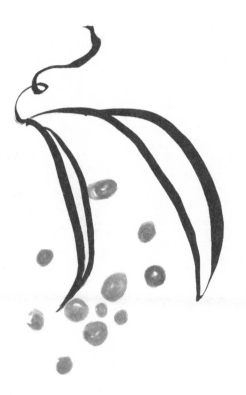

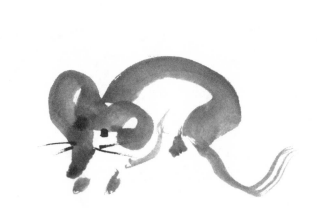

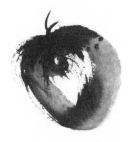

*Charlotte Selver loves to remind her students that "Every moment is a moment."
There is something liberating about this statement. Every moment is new and un-
precedented. It is filled with possibilities.*

*Can you feel this as you are walking? Can each step be invigorated with this
sense of newness? Can you be surprised by the taste of an orange or a sip of tea? Can
you make spaghetti sauce as if it were the first time, although you've made it a thousand times before?*

*One of my favorite Zen stories is about a man who was chased by a ferocious tiger.
The man ran to the edge of a cliff where he grabbed hold of a vine and swung himself
over the side. Still hanging from the vine, he breathed a deep sigh of relief, thinking
he was saved.*

*But looking up, he saw the tiger waiting for him. Looking down into the ravine
below, he saw another tiger waiting for him. He looked around and saw two tiny
mice begin to chew away at the vine.*

*Growing on the side of the cliff next to him was a beautiful ripe strawberry. He
could smell its fragrance. It looked like a jewel glinting in the sunshine. Reaching
out, he gently picked it and took a small bite, savoring its essence. How sweet it
tasted!*

*What freedom this story conveys! Although the man is in a terrible situation, he
is undaunted. Glimmering in front of him is a strawberry, and he eats it as if he
had no other care in the world.*

Salads

Every day our markets are filled with new kinds of lettuces, fresh herbs, and greens. All have different tastes and textures. There are the soft butter lettuces, the colorful red oak leaf, the crispy romaine, and the frilly leafed lettuces. A mixture of different colors and shapes looks wonderful in a large wooden salad bowl. Various greens mixed with lettuce add contrast and flavor. Arugula and watercress are peppery. Sorrel has a lemony flavor. Curly endive and red radicchio have a mild bitterness.

Salads can be simple with just a butter lettuce and a mustard honey dressing. Or they can be much more complicated and fanciful. Green leaf salads can include cooked beans or lentils, toasted sunflower seeds, and roasted nuts. Try some new ingredients like jicama from Mexico. It is crisp, cool, and sweet in salads. Or toss in some grilled tofu. Make a salad with marinated vegetables or sautéed shiitake mushrooms.

Salad dressings can be complicated with all sorts of nut oils, flavored vinegars, and different herbs and spices. But I find, as in most cooking, that the simplest is the best.

Use the best quality extra virgin olive oil in your dressings. One of the most delicious salads I ever had was in an Italian restaurant that served a dressing made with only extra virgin olive oil and a touch of fresh lemon juice. With delicate salads, make a similar dressing so the tastes of the lettuces can shine. If the salad is heartier with steamed vegetables, use a flavorful dressing such as Ewa's Honey Mustard Dressing (page 166) or Chili Lime Basil Dressing (page 167).

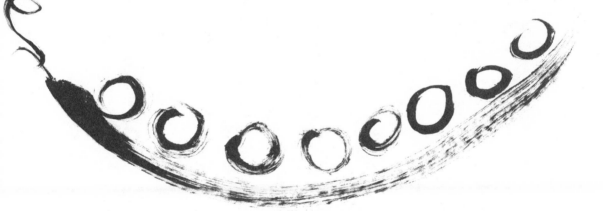

PEAS ON EARTH

Mesclun *Salad*

8 cups (about) mixed lettuce such as red
    leaf or oak leaf

1 cup each curly endive, arugula, and
    red radicchio

6 tablespoons extra virgin olive oil

1 tablespoon lemon juice

Salt

Freshly ground pepper

SERVES 4 TO 6

Mesclun is a Provençal term for a salad mixture of young tender lettuces and greens. The mingling of colors, textures, and contrasting flavors are the highlight of the salad, so use a very simple dressing. Extra virgin olive oil and a light sprinkling of fresh lemon juice is perfect.

Mesclun mix has become very popular. A big basket of it is now offered not only in my local market but also in the big chain supermarkets. It's expensive, but there's nothing to compare with such a fresh and delicate salad.

Wash and dry the lettuces and greens. Tear them into bite-size pieces and place in a large salad bowl.

In a small bowl, combine the oil and lemon juice. Add the salt and freshly ground pepper to taste.

Toss the lettuces and greens with just enough dressing to lightly coat the salad.

Mixed Green Salad with Aduki Beans

Beans readily absorb the flavors of oil and vinegar, and are a good way to include them in your meals. Nuts add crunch as well as flavor.

Wash and dry the spinach and lettuce. Tear into bite-size pieces and place in a large salad bowl with the cabbage, beans, and onion. Just before serving, toss with enough dressing to lightly coat the salad. Garnish with croutons or toasted nuts.

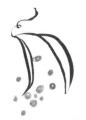

1 bunch spinach (3/4 pound)

4 cups (about) oak leaf lettuce

2 cups thinly sliced white cabbage

1 cup cooked and cooled aduki beans

1/2 cup thinly sliced red onion

Ewa's Honey Mustard Dressing (page 166)

Croutons or toasted nuts, for garnish

SERVES 4 TO 6

Croutons
Delicious in salads, croutons are crunchy and flavorful. The best croutons are made from dry French bread. Cut the bread into cubes. Heat 1 tablespoon of butter or olive oil in a large frying pan. Add the bread and cook over medium heat, until browned on all sides. Season with salt and pepper.

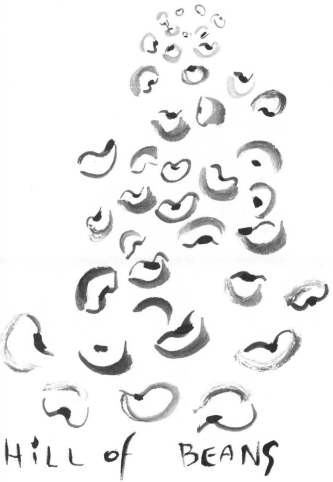

HiLL of BEANS

Mixed Greens with Zucchini, Red Pepper, and Sunflower Seeds

1 head romaine lettuce (about 3/4 pound)

2 cups arugula or curly endive

2 small zucchini, finely grated

1 medium red pepper, chopped

Orange Raspberry Vinaigrette (page 167)

1/2 cup toasted sunflower seeds

SERVES 4 TO 6

Green leaf salads look beautiful with a few thinly grated and sliced vegetables.

Wash and dry the lettuce and greens. Place in a large salad bowl. Just before serving, toss with the zucchini, red pepper, and just enough dressing to lightly coat all the ingredients. Garnish with the toasted sunflower seeds.

Carrot and Navy Bean Mixed Salad

1 cup sliced carrots

3/4 pound oak leaf lettuce

1 cup arugula or curly endive

2 cups thinly sliced red cabbage

3/4 cup cooked navy beans

Basic Olive Oil Dressing (page 166)

SERVES 4 TO 6

When you are looking for a colorful and hearty salad, this is the one to try.

Steam the carrots and set aside to cool. Wash and dry the lettuce and greens. Slice the red cabbage as thinly as possible. Just before serving, toss all the ingredients with just enough dressing to lightly coat the salad.

Broccoli Salad with Tofu and Chili Lime Basil Dressing

This is a good salad to serve with a light soup or a simple cous-cous pilaf.

Steam the broccoli for 5 minutes, until it is cooked al dente and bright green. Remove from the heat and immediately rinse under cold water. Drain and place in a large salad bowl with the tofu. Toss with half the dressing and marinate for ½ hour. Just before serving, add the romaine and toss with just enough dressing to lightly cover the lettuce. Garnish with croutons.

1½ cups broccoli florets

2 cups Stir-Fry Tofu (page 133)

½ cup Chili Lime Basil Dressing (page 167)

¾ pound romaine lettuce

Toasted croutons, for garnish

SERVES 4

Jicama and Avocado Salad

Sweet jicama, flavored with tart raspberry vinegar, is delectable with avocados. Serve this salad with crisp tacos.

Wash the lettuce and dry it. Tear it into bite-size pieces and place in a large salad bowl. Peel the jicama and cut into julienne strips. Just before serving, cut the avocados in half, remove the pits, and peel. Place face down and cut into thin slices. Toss all the ingredients with the raspberry dressing. Add enough dressing to generously coat the ingredients.

Heat the oven to 350 degrees and bake the tacos for 10 minutes, until crisp.

Serve the salad on individual plates. Break the tacos in half and place them sticking out of the sides of the salad.

1 head red leaf lettuce (about ¾ pound)

¾ pound jicama

2 ripe avocados

Orange Raspberry Vinaigrette (page 167)

4–6 tacos or tostadas

SERVES 4 TO 6

Thai Carrot Salad with Peanuts

CHILI VINAIGRETTE:

¼ cup rice vinegar

3 tablespoons fresh lime juice

1 tablespoon fresh orange juice

1 tablespoon grated orange zest

1 tablespoon chopped fresh cilantro

3 tablespoons pure maple syrup

¼ teaspoon red chili flakes

3 cups grated carrots

1 cup chopped peanuts

Finely chopped fresh mint, for garnish

SERVES 4

I first tasted this salad in a Thai restaurant where it was served with grilled salmon. It was so delicious I decided to invent my own, using the flavors of fresh cilantro, limes, mint, peanuts, and hot chilis. Be careful with the chili flakes—this salad can get too hot!

In a food processor, blend all the vinaigrette ingredients. Add the chili flakes last, adding them a little at a time to taste.

Wash the carrots with a brush and grate into a large bowl. Add half the dressing, saving the rest for another use. (It will keep, refrigerated, for up to 1 week.) Marinate the salad for 15 to 20 minutes before serving. Garnish with chopped peanuts and mint.

Tofu Salad

Color makes this salad, and fresh herbs and lemon give it flavor. Lovage is wonderful here, but if it isn't available use fresh basil or cilantro. If you season the salad with cilantro, include ¼ cup minced Anaheim or poblano chili peppers with the rest of the ingredients.

Try other vegetables with the tofu: Red and green peppers, shredded red radicchio, or purple and green cabbage are lovely.

The tofu should be as fresh as possible. Rinse it under cold water and drain in a colander for ½ hour. Using a potato masher or a large fork, mash the tofu with the oil, lemon juice, cayenne, and tamari. It should have the consistency of cottage cheese.

In a large salad bowl, gently mix all the vegetables and fresh herbs with the tofu. Taste for seasoning and add more herbs, lemon juice, and freshly ground pepper as needed. Refrigerate for an hour before serving, arrange on a serving platter with fresh greens.

2 10-ounce blocks firm tofu

4 tablespoons canola oil

1 tablespoon fresh lemon juice

Pinch of cayenne

3 tablespoons tamari

¾ cup diced zucchini

¾ cup diced yellow summer squash

2 stalks celery, fined sliced

1 cup bite-size pieces string beans

2 tablespoons finely chopped fresh
    lovage, basil, or cilantro

Freshly ground pepper

8 to 10 leaves romaine or red leaf
    lettuce, for serving

SERVES 4

Mediterranean Green Salad

8 cups (about) red leaf lettuce

2 large Idaho baking potatoes, baked,
   cooled, and cut into bite-size pieces

$^{1}/_{4}$ cup grated Parmesan cheese

$^{1}/_{2}$ cup pitted and halved black olives

$^{1}/_{4}$ cup extra virgin olive oil

1 tablespoon balsamic vinegar or more to
   taste

Salt

Freshly ground pepper

SERVES 4 TO 6

Balsamic vinegar, Parmesan cheese, and olives bring a hint of the Mediterranean to this salad of potatoes and tender red leaf lettuce.

Wash and dry the lettuce. Tear the leaves into bite-size pieces and place in a large salad bowl. Add the potatoes, Parmesan cheese, and olives.

In a separate bowl, whisk the olive oil and vinegar together. Season to taste with salt and freshly ground pepper. Toss with the salad, taste for seasoning, and serve.

Lentil Salad

This is one of my favorite salads. The earthy flavor of the lentils is enhanced by marinating them with fresh herbs, garlic, and sweet balsamic vinegar. The tofu absorbs the flavors of the marinade, creating a salad of contrasting textures, colors, and tastes.

Rinse the lentils. Place them with the bay leaf in a medium pot and cover generously with water. Bring to a simmer, partially cover with a lid, and cook for 20 to 30 minutes, until al dente. The lentils should be firm and hold their shape. After simmering for 10 minutes, stir in the diced carrots.

Wash the tofu and set aside to drain.

Prepare the dressing. Place the garlic and salt in a small wooden bowl. Using the back of a spoon or a pestle, press the garlic to a paste. Mix in the balsamic vinegar, olive oil, and tamari.

When the lentils are cooked, drain and immediately toss in a large bowl with the dressing. Gently mix in three-quarters of the cubed tofu and red onion. Set aside to marinate for 1 hour.

Before serving, toss in the fresh herbs and parsley. Season to taste with freshly ground pepper. Add a touch more balsamic vinegar if needed. Break the rest of the tofu into tiny pieces, scatter on top of the salad, sprinkle with paprika, and serve.

1 ½ cups dried lentils

1 bay leaf

1 carrot, diced

10 ounces firm tofu, cubed

4 garlic cloves, minced

⅛ teaspoon salt

3 tablespoons balsamic vinegar

¼ cup olive oil

1 tablespoon tamari

½ medium red onion, minced

2 tablespoons minced fresh lovage

2 tablespoons minced fresh sage

½ cup chopped fresh parsley

Freshly ground pepper

Paprika

SERVES 4

Marinated Tomatoes

6 ripe tomatoes (about 1 ½ pounds)

3 garlic cloves, minced

⅛ teaspoon salt

¼ cup extra virgin olive oil

3 tablespoons balsamic vinegar

Finely chopped fresh herbs: ¼ cup basil
    and 2 tablespoons lovage

Freshly ground pepper

Fresh parsley or basil, for garnish

SERVES 4

This is a summer dish and, of course, the fresher and sweeter the tomatoes, the better. This salad goes well with slices of smoked mozzarella and fresh baked French bread.

Cut the tomatoes in half and then in ¼-inch slices. Lay in a shallow pan.

Place the garlic and salt in a small bowl or mortar. Using the back of a spoon or a pestle, mash the garlic until it becomes a paste. Stir in the oil, vinegar, and fresh herbs. Season to taste with freshly ground pepper.

Pour this marinade over the tomatoes and refrigerate for at least 2 hours, turning the tomatoes every so often. The juices will become incredibly sweet and garlicky. When serving, lift the tomatoes out of the marinade with a slotted spoon. Place on a plate and serve garnished with fresh basil leaves. Save the marinade for up to 1 week in the refrigerator. Use it as a marinade for grilled vegetables or tofu.

Crunchy celery, fresh dill, and lots of parsley give this salad its character. It's beautiful with pale red and green colors.

In a large pot, cover the potatoes with water and cook over medium heat for 10 to 15 minutes: The potatoes should be soft but still hold their shape in the salad.

While the potatoes are cooking, make the dressing. In a small bowl or mortar, using the back of a spoon or a pestle, press the garlic with the salt to form a paste. Stir in the olive oil, vinegar, and mustard.

When the potatoes are cooked, drain them. Place in a large bowl and immediately toss them with the dressing. Stir in the celery, onion, parsley, dill, and Parmesan cheese. Season to taste with freshly ground pepper and a pinch of cayenne. Allow to cool before serving.

6 cups new red potatoes (about 1 ½ pounds), cut into bite-size pieces

3 large garlic cloves, minced

¼ teaspoon salt

¼ cup olive oil

3 tablespoons balsamic vinegar

3 teaspoons Dijon mustard

2 cups thinly sliced celery

½ large red onion, chopped

½ cup chopped fresh parsley

2 tablespoons minced fresh dill

½ cup grated Parmesan cheese

Freshly ground pepper

Pinch of cayenne

SERVES 4

Thai Noodle Salad

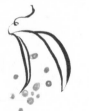

8 ounces soba noodles

2 large handfuls spinach or 4 cups with
  stems discarded

3 cups mung bean sprouts

1/2 red pepper, finely chopped

2 tablespoons finely chopped fresh mint

1/4 to 1/2 cup Chili Lime Basil Dressing
  (page 167)

Mint sprigs, for garnish

SERVES 4

This is a light refreshing salad accentuated by the tastes of basil, mint, and chili. The coffee color of the soba noodles looks beautiful with the deep green of spinach.

Bring a large pot of water to a full boil. Add a tiny bit of oil and cook the soba noodles for 5 minutes, until al dente. Rinse under cold water, drain, and set aside in a large salad bowl.

Wash the spinach, discard the stems, and pat dry. Break into bite-size pieces. Toss the noodles with the spinach, mung sprouts, red pepper, and mint. Carefully mix all the ingredients together with the lime dressing. Garnish with sprigs of mint.

Cajun Coleslaw

This is a wonderful version of coleslaw, refreshing with jicama and delicate fennel. The lemon and cayenne make it spicy and tart, while the caramelized walnuts add a hint of sweet.

Place the jicama in a large mixing bowl with the rest of the ingredients. Toss well with the Cajun Dressing. Chill in the refrigerator for 1 hour before serving.

CARAMELIZED WALNUTS
The recipes in this book rarely use sugar, but in this case there is no substitute for making caramel.

1/4 cup sugar

1/4 cup water

1 1/2 cups walnuts

Combine the sugar and water in a medium-size skillet. Cook over medium heat. Do not stir, but swirl the pan by the handle to dissolve the sugar. When the liquid becomes clear, it will start to bubble. Cook for 5 minutes, until the bubbles are thick and heavy. The syrup may begin to look caramel brown. Toss in the walnuts and stir them in the syrup until all the liquid is gone. Immediately spread the walnuts on a cookie sheet to cool. Store in an airtight container until serving.

2 cups peeled and julienned jicama (about 10 ounces)

1 cup thinly sliced red cabbage

1 cup julienned carrots

1 cup julienned fennel bulb

1/2 cup coarsely chopped Caramelized Walnuts

1/2 cup Cajun Dressing (page 167)

SERVES 4

Broccoli, Shiitake, and Tomato Salad

10 shiitake mushrooms

1 tablespoon butter

1 tablespoon lemon juice

3 garlic cloves, minced

⅛ teaspoon salt

¼ cup olive oil

3 tablespoons balsamic vinegar

Freshly ground pepper

4 ripe tomatoes

¼ cup chopped fresh basil

1 head broccoli (about 1 pound)

Parsley or shredded purple cabbage, for garnish

SERVES 4

Broccoli, fresh tomatoes, garlic, and fragrant basil go well with shiitake mushrooms that have been sautéed in butter and lemon. Fresh shiitakes are best, but if they're unavailable use dried ones or substitute dried porcinis.

If you are using dried mushrooms, soak them in water for ½ hour. When they are soft, drain and save the stems for soup stock. Finely slice the caps. Heat the butter in a small skillet. Cook the mushrooms over medium heat for 10–15 minutes, stirring frequently. Stir in the lemon juice and set aside.

To make the dressing, place the garlic and salt in a small bowl or mortar. Using the back of a spoon or a pestle, press the garlic into a paste. Stir in the oil and vinegar. Season to taste with freshly ground pepper.

Core the tomatoes and cut into bite-size pieces. Place in a large mixing bowl and toss with the basil and mushrooms.

Divide the broccoli into florets of equal size, 2 to 3 inches long. Trim the stalks by cutting off the ends and peeling the thick skin with a paring knife. Slice the stems into bite-size pieces.

Steam the broccoli until just tender, about 5 minutes. It will turn bright green. Immediately plunge into cold water. Drain well and mix with the tomatoes and mushrooms. Stir in the dressing and marinate for at least 1 hour. Taste to adjust the seasoning. Garnish with parsley or shredded purple cabbage.

Zucchini Salad

This simple salad allows the tender fragrance of the zucchini to shine. There are two keys to this salad. The first is to use the finest aged Parmesan cheese, Parmegiana Reggiano. The second is to julienne the zucchini. Prepared in this way, the zucchini make beautiful patterns and colors on the plate.

8 medium zucchini

1 tablespoon olive oil

2 medium garlic cloves, minced

1 tablespoon butter

1/2 cup slivered almonds

Salt

Freshly ground pepper

Parmegiana Reggiano

Finely chopped fresh parsley, for garnish

SERVES 4

Cut the zucchini in 3-inch-long slices and then into thin julienne.

Heat the oil in a skillet. Add the garlic and julienned zucchini and cook over medium heat for 3 to 4 minutes, stirring frequently. The zucchini should be half cooked.

Heat the butter in a separate pan. Briefly brown the almonds over medium heat. Place in a large bowl and toss with the zucchini. Season to taste with salt and freshly ground pepper.

Serve warm, arranged on individual serving plates. Top with shavings of Parmesan cheese and garnish with chopped parsley.

Avocado and Red Peppers

I can think of no other salad as elegant and colorful as this one.

Cut the avocados in half, remove the seeds, and peel. Place the avocados face down and cut into thin slices.

Place the slices on a serving plate or individual plates. Top with red pepper relish and garnish with cilantro.

2 ripe avocados

1 ⅓ cups Red Pepper Relish (page 168)

Finely chopped fresh cilantro, for garnish

SERVES 4

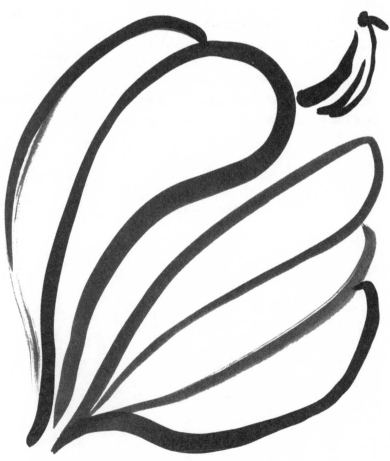

Pear, Jicama, and Beet Salad

In Mexico, jicama is often sprinkled with chili powder and lime juice or combined with oranges and cilantro. This colorful salad highlights the contrasting flavors of jicama, fresh ripe pears, and sweet beets. Serve on a bed of crisp lettuce and greens.

Peel the beets and cut them into julienne strips. Steam for 10 minutes, until soft. Drain and cool to room temperature. Place the cubed jicama in a bowl and marinate with lemon juice for 30 minutes. Core the pears and cut into thin slices. If you slice them in advance of serving, toss with some lemon juice so they don't brown. In a dry skillet, lightly toast the walnuts for 5 minutes over medium heat, stirring frequently. Coarsely chop them.

Wash and dry the lettuces and greens.

To arrange the salad, place the greens on individual salad plates. Arrange ½ pear per person in a circle on top of the greens. Place the beets around the pears, with the jicama mounded in the center. Scatter with the toasted walnuts and drizzle the salad dressing on top.

3 medium beets

1 cup peeled and cubed jicama (about 5 ounces)

1 tablespoon lemon juice

2 ripe pears

½ cup walnuts

4 cups mixed garden lettuces

1 cup watercress or arugula

Ewa's Honey Mustard Dressing (page 166)

MAKES 4 SMALL INDIVIDUAL SALADS

Sauces and Salad Dressings

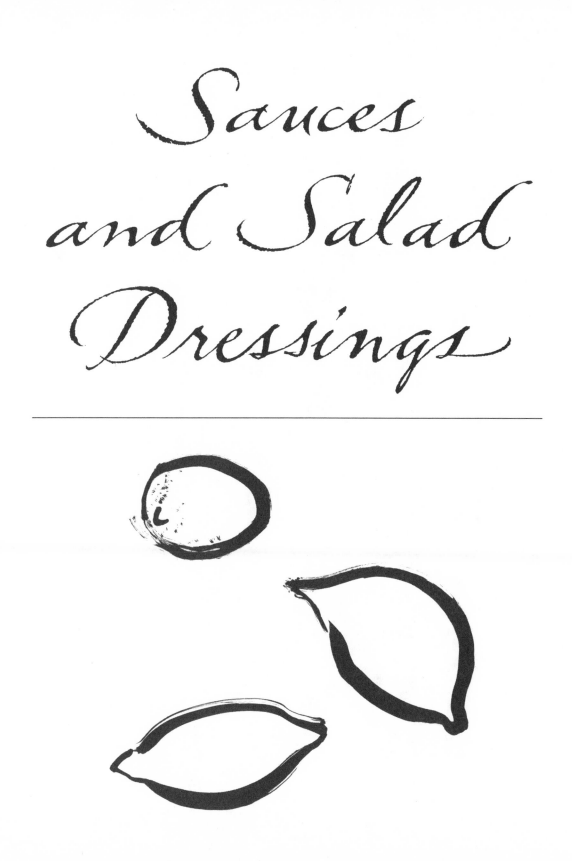

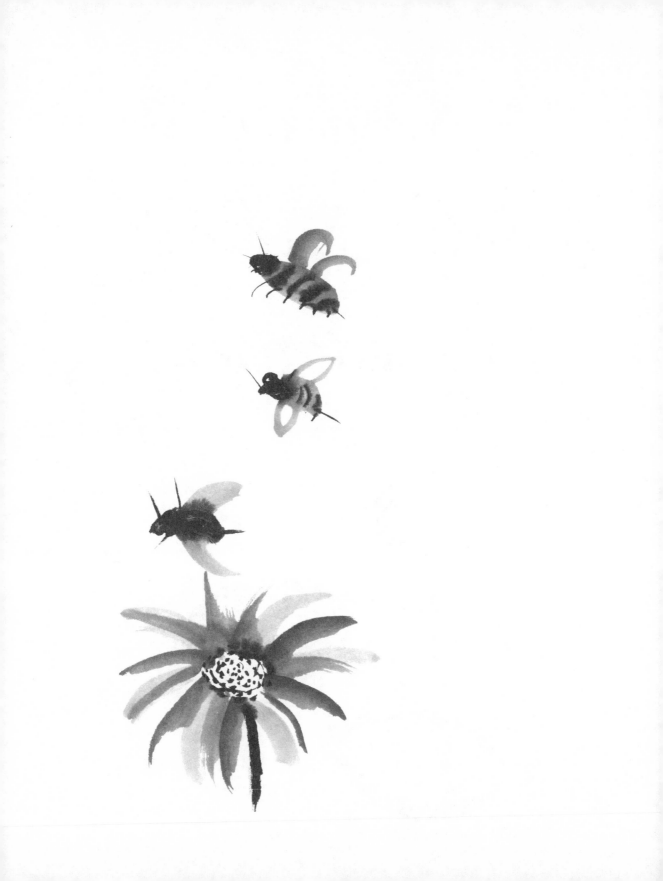

When we first bring our awareness to breathing or to small everyday actions, we may notice that it's hard to stay with it. We are easily distracted. But with practice, this restlessness will soon disappear.

Any activity—whether you are cooking a meal, walking to the grocery store, or having tea with friends—can be an occasion to practice being mindful, attentive to what happens in the moment.

The next time you set the table for dinner, try this out.

As you fold each napkin, feel what first becomes conscious to you. Are your hands awake to the softness of the paper or the texture of the cloth?

When you pick up a plate, notice how you hold it. How heavy is it?

When you put it down, can you feel the first instant when it touches the table? Find the moment when the table takes the full weight of the plate and you are no longer holding it.

Practice this with forks, knives, and spoons of different weights, or your best wineglasses. Take your time to feel what happens. Savor the taste of it.

You may become aware of all sorts of sensations. What happens in your breathing?

What do you notice about the way you are standing? Feel how your balance changes as you reach to put the dishes down on the table.

What do you discover? Every moment brings us something new to relate to—the meals we prepare, the ground upon which we stand, the air which we breathe, the people we are with. Everything we do, everything we meet has the potential to bring us into a closer relationship with the world around us.

Sauces and Salad Dressings

If your cooking repertoire were to include only a good soup and a good sauce, you would be well ahead of the game.

The basic cream sauces, which the French have mastered, are easy to create once you have learned how to make the basic roux. A Béchamel Sauce can add elegance and taste to a plate of simple steamed vegetables or crepes.

Brush Spicy Sesame Butter or Cilantro Pesto on broiled or grilled vegetables and tofu. Make your own Apricot Lime Chutney and serve it alongside Curry Pilaf with Chickpeas and Couscous.

Basic Tomato Sauce and Sweet Red Sauce are delicious on pastas or rice, and the Asian flavors of lime, ginger, and cilantro, whether in a salad dressing or in a sauce, make a meal special.

Basic Tomato Sauce

An old Italian man I know calls his tomato sauce "gravy." It is the most important part of his family's Sunday meal. His wife spends hours making it. This version takes far less time. Perhaps it's not as rich, but it's every bit as delicious. Make a fair amount and keep the extra in the refrigerator or freezer. It provides the basis for many delicious recipes.

Heat the oil in a saucepan. Add the garlic and onions and cook over high heat for 3 to 4 minutes, stirring frequently. After a minute of cooking, add the bay leaf and herbs. When the onions begin to look translucent, stir in the tomatoes, cook for another minute, and add the water. Simmer for 1 hour, partially covered. Season with tamari, salt, and freshly ground pepper.

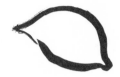

1 tablespoon olive oil

3 medium garlic cloves, minced

1 large yellow onion, chopped

1 bay leaf

1 tablespoon dried basil

¼ teaspoon dried oregano

3½ cups chopped tomatoes or 1 28-ounce can crushed tomatoes

1 cup water

1 tablespoon tamari

Salt

Freshly ground pepper

MAKES 4 CUPS SAUCE

Sweet Red Sauce

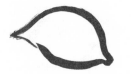

The sweetness of carrots, red peppers, and acorn squash blend perfectly with the flavors of tomatoes, garlic, and olive oil. Try this sauce as a topping for pizza or polenta, in crepes, or simply served over rice.

Cut the acorn squash in half and scoop out the seeds and strings. Place it face down and cut into ⅓-inch-thick slices. Cut these in half for bite-size pieces.

Heat the olive oil in a large pot. Sauté the garlic and onion over high heat for 3 to 4 minutes, stirring frequently. After a minute of cooking, add the herbs. When the onions become translucent, stir in the carrots and squash. Cook for 2 or 3 minutes over high heat. Lower the flame and stir in the tomatoes and water. Cover and simmer until the vegetables are soft, about 30 minutes.

Stir in the red peppers and cook for 5 minutes. The peppers should still have color and crunch. Season with tamari, salt, and freshly ground pepper to taste. Garnish with parsley.

½ pound acorn squash (1¾ to 2 cups sliced squash)

2 tablespoons olive oil

3 medium garlic cloves, minced

1 large yellow onion, chopped

1 tablespoon dried basil

1 tablespoon dried marjoram

2 carrots cut into bite-size pieces

2 medium tomatoes, chopped

¼ cup water

2 red peppers, sliced

2 tablespoons tamari

Salt

Freshly ground pepper

Finely chopped fresh parsley, for garnish

MAKES 6 CUPS SAUCE

Béchamel Sauce

This is a luscious cream sauce flavored lightly with tamari and sesame butter. It is delicious on crepes, zucchini fritters, plain rice, and steamed vegetables.

In The Beat'n Path Cafe we used to trade dinners for all our plumbing work. Our plumber's favorite dish was a plate of beans, rice, and sautéed vegetables covered with this béchamel sauce. It was so popular that we finally named it "The Plumber's Special," and it became an established part of our cafe menu.

Heat the oil in a heavy saucepan over medium heat. Tablespoon by tablespoon, mix enough flour into the oil to make a paste. This is the roux. Cook for 5 minutes over low heat, stirring frequently. When the flour seems to be browning, and it smells nutty, slowly whisk in the hot water. Add enough water to create a thick sauce. Stir in the tahini, tamari, and freshly ground pepper. Mix well and serve immediately.

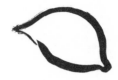

3 tablespoons canola oil

4 ½ tablespoons whole wheat pastry flour

1 to 2 cups hot water

2 tablespoons tahini

1 ½ tablespoons tamari

Freshly ground pepper

MAKES 1 ¾ CUPS SAUCE

Pesto

2 cups (closely packed) fresh basil leaves

$^1/_3$ cup olive oil

$^1/_4$ cup water

$^1/_4$ cup chopped walnuts

3 small garlic cloves, minced

$^1/_2$ cup freshly grated Parmesan cheese

Salt

Freshly ground pepper to taste

MAKES I CUP

Pesto is wonderful to make in the summer when there is an abundance of basil. Serve with fresh pasta or as a topping on sautéed tofu. It's great on pizzas or as a sauce with steamed vegetables.

Wash the fresh basil leaves and pat dry. In a food processor, blend all the ingredients until smooth. Add salt and freshly ground pepper to taste.

Variation: Parsley Pesto

We could never grow basil in the garden at Dai Bosatsu Zendo, so we substituted parsley for the fresh basil. Parsley is rich in vitamins and minerals, and it makes a wonderful, nutritious sauce. The recipe is the same as for Pesto.

Cilantro Pesto

2 cups closely packed fresh cilantro

1 teaspoon chopped serrano chili

1 garlic clove, chopped

$^1/_4$ cup walnuts

$^1/_2$ cup grated Parmesan cheese

1 teaspoon lime juice

$^1/_4$ cup olive oil

$^1/_4$ cup water

MAKES I CUP

Once you discover the delights of fresh cilantro, you will find yourself including it in all your favorite recipes. Try this pesto on top of Broiled Tomatoes (page 121) or as a topping on a Mexican-style pizza.

Wash the cilantro and pat dry. In a food processor, blend all the ingredients together until smooth.

Asian-Style Peanut Sauce

I love the Asian combinations of lime, cilantro, mint, peanuts, and hot chili. Serve this sauce over steamed vegetables for a Thai-style dinner or as a dipping sauce for Vietnamese Spring Rolls (page 101). If you like it hot, add more chili peppers.

Wash the cilantro and pat dry. Add all the ingredients into a food processor and blend until smooth.

¼ cup chopped fresh cilantro
¾ cup peanut butter
2 tablespoons chopped fresh mint
¼ teaspoon hot chili pepper flakes
1 cup water
4 tablespoons lime juice

MAKES 1¾ CUPS SAUCE

Cashew Ginger Sauce

The zesty flavors of ginger and lime balance the sweetness of cashews. This sauce goes very well with hot steamed vegetables or tossed with fettuccine. It is also an excellent substitute for sour cream in stroganoffs.

In a dry skillet, toast the cashews over medium heat for 5 minutes, tossing continually to prevent burning.

Peel and grate the ginger. Either in a towel or your hands, squeeze the juice from the grated ginger into a food processor. Add all the ingredients except the water into the food processor and blend until smooth and creamy. Continue to blend while adding the water a little at a time.

1 cup cashews
3 inches ginger
¼ cup canola oil
2 medium garlic cloves, minced
2 tablespoons tamari
1 tablespoon chopped fresh cilantro
Juice of 1 lime
¾ cup hot water

MAKES 1½ CUPS SAUCE

Ewa's Honey Mustard Dressing

Juice of 1 lemon
1 teaspoon clover honey
1 teaspoon Dijon mustard
¼ cup extra virgin olive oil
Salt
Freshly ground pepper

MAKES ½ CUP DRESSING

My friend Ewa didn't invent this dressing, but she did teach me how to make it and since then it has become my favorite. I always make twice as much as I need and keep the unused portion in the refrigerator. This thick and creamy dressing keeps for up to ten days.

Combine all the ingredients in either a bowl or a jar with a tight-fitting lid. It's easier to shake the jar than to whisk the ingredients in a bowl, but either method is fine. Season to taste with salt and freshly ground pepper.

Basic Olive Oil Dressing

3 medium garlic cloves, minced
½ teaspoon salt
¼ cup extra virgin olive oil
2 tablespoons balsamic vinegar
Freshly ground pepper

MAKES ⅓ CUP DRESSING

My mother has been making this dressing for as long as I can remember. She puts her own special magic in it which I have never quite been able to capture. She also uses enormous amounts of garlic, salt, and pepper. Here is the version I have good luck with.

Put the minced garlic in a small bowl. Add the salt and, using the back of a spoon or a wooden pestle, press the garlic until it becomes like a paste. Add a small amount of oil and mix very well. Add the rest of the oil and the vinegar. Season with quite a bit of freshly ground pepper and more salt to taste.

Chili Lime Basil Dressing

This dressing is a perfect complement to a meal of Thai flavors. Use it as a marinade for tofu or as a sauce for grilled shish kebabs. If fresh Anaheim chilis are unavailable, use canned chili peppers.

Wash the basil and pat dry. In a food processor, blend all the ingredients together until creamy and smooth. If you want a spicier dressing, add more red chili peppers, but be careful, they are very hot.

½ cup tightly packed basil leaves
2 tablespoons fresh lime juice
2 medium garlic cloves, minced
2 tablespoons minced Anaheim chili peppers
⅓ cup canola oil
1 teaspoon clover honey
Pinch of crushed red pepper flakes
Salt

MAKES ½ CUP DRESSING

Cajun Dressing

Sometimes there is just no substitute for mayonnaise. Spicy with cayenne, this makes a perfect dressing for Cajun Coleslaw (page 151) or a potato salad. Try it as a dip with crudités.

Blend all the ingredients. Add more cayenne or lemon juice according to your taste.

1 cup mayonnaise
Juice of 1 large lemon
1 teaspoon clover honey
1½ teaspoons cayenne

MAKES ⅔ CUP DRESSING

Orange Raspberry Vinaigrette

It's worth having walnut oil and raspberry vinegar on hand. This is a delightful dressing, great to serve on cold soba noodles in the summer.

Combine all the ingredients in a jar with a tight lid. Shake well and serve.

½ cup orange juice
⅓ cup walnut, canola, or olive oil
¼ cup raspberry vinegar
1 tablespoon lime juice

MAKES 1 CUP DRESSING

Red Pepper Relish

2 medium red peppers

½ cup finely chopped red onion

1 large garlic clove, minced

½ cup olive oil

2 tablespoons balsamic vinegar

1 teaspoon tamari

Salt

Freshly ground pepper

MAKES 1 ⅓ CUPS

Red peppers are sweet and rich in vitamin C. Their vibrant color makes them wonderful to use as a garnish and great for vegetable sautés and salads. This relish is simple and quick to make. Serve it over slices of avocado or as a topping for zucchini fritters or crepes.

Cut the peppers in half and remove the seeds, veins, and stems. Cut them into large pieces. Coarsely blend for a minute or two in a food processor with the rest of the ingredients. Don't make a paste. Season to taste with salt and freshly ground pepper.

Apricot Lime Chutney

1 ⅓ cups finely chopped dried apricots

3 fresh jalapeño chili peppers, minced

½ teaspoon cumin powder

3 tablespoons lime juice

MAKES 2 CUPS

Put the apricots in a medium-size saucepan with enough water to just cover them. Simmer for 20 minutes, until soft. Drain and combine them in a mixing bowl with the rest of the ingredients. Cool before serving. The chutney will keep in the refrigerator for a week.

East West Salsa

Made with fresh chili peppers and Japanese pickled ginger, this salsa is refreshing and delicious when served as a topping on chilled soba noodles. If you like it very hot, add crushed red chili peppers or cayenne.

In a mixing bowl, combine all the ingredients. Season to taste with salt and freshly ground pepper. Let the salsa sit for an hour before serving. It will keep in the refrigerator for up to 2 days.

1 Anaheim chili pepper, seeded and minced

2 jalapeño chili peppers, seeded and minced

½ red pepper, finely chopped

3 tablespoons minced Japanese gari (pickled ginger)

2 scallions, finely sliced

1 tablespoon lemon juice

Salt

Freshly ground pepper

MAKES 1 ½ CUPS

Spicy Sesame Butter

This light sesame butter can be as spicy and hot as you like by just adding more or less cayenne. Serve it as a topping on grilled Japanese eggplant. Make it into a sauce and serve with steamed or roasted vegetables or as a dressing in pita sandwiches stuffed with fresh vegetables.

To make the sesame butter, in a food processor, blend the tahini, garlic, olive oil, and lemon juice until smooth and creamy. Add cayenne to taste, ¼ teaspoon makes a very hot dressing!

For the sesame dressing, add water and tamari to the rest of the ingredients and blend in a food processor until creamy. Season with salt to taste.

4 tablespoons tahini

2 small garlic cloves, minced

2 tablespoons olive oil

2 tablespoons lemon juice

¼ teaspoon cayenne

½ cup water

1 teaspoon tamari

Salt

MAKES 1 CUP

Breakfast Ideas

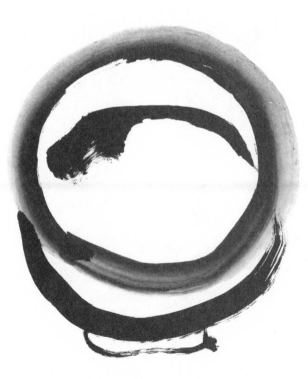

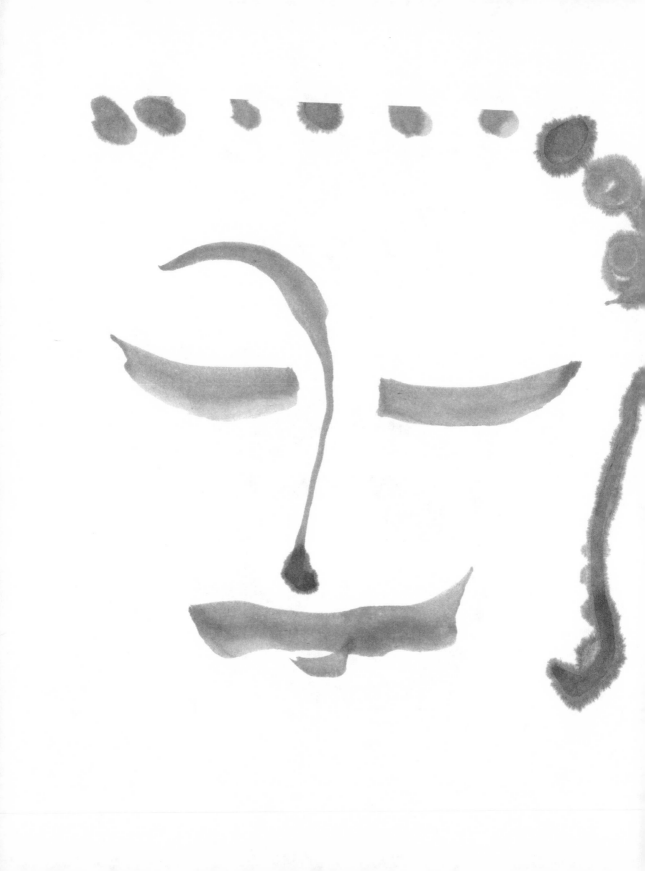

The great Zen master Hakuin Zenji said that "Everyday mind is the Way." Cooking a meal, waiting for the bus, gardening—any activity can be the Way.

In every moment of attention our minds are concentrated. It's as simple as reaching for a glass of water and feeling what happens in that small movement. It's as simple as becoming aware of our breathing or noticing each step we take as we walk down the street.

When we are focused this way we become quiet and peaceful. Our awareness becomes like a still lake. When a pebble is tossed into a lake, the water ripples outward in circles that grow wider and wider until they finally disappear. The lake becomes quiet again.

We are like this lake. When our mind is quiet we can see and feel things with deeper clarity. We see how all phenomena arise and pass away, just like ripples appearing and disappearing in the water. We recognize the momentariness of life and experience its spaciousness and profound resonance.

The simple tasks of cooking can lead to deep understanding. Just washing the lettuce or stirring the soup. Just going from place to place in the kitchen. Kneading the bread or oiling the bread pan. Every moment is precious.

> If your ears see,
> And eyes hear
> Not a doubt you'll cherish—
> How naturally the rain drips
> From the eaves!
> DAITO KOKUSHI
> (FOURTEENTH CENTURY)

Breakfast Ideas

The aroma of fresh brewed coffee and warmth of muffins right out of the oven welcomes us first thing in the morning. Hot oatmeal in the winter or fresh fruit salads and granola in the summer can start our day.

Breakfast can be as simple as a piece of toast or as elaborate as the imagination can make it. We often serve breakfast buffet style at the guest house at Dai Bosatsu, and it's everyone's favorite meal. The serving table is laden with platters of freshly sliced fruit, plates of crepes or pancakes, a casserole of spoon bread, and baskets of hot muffins. Sometimes the guests gather in the kitchen waiting for the next pancakes hot off the griddle.

The air outside is fresh with the smell of flowers and the lake sparkles in the morning sunshine.

Surprise Pancakes

This is a favorite breakfast surprise. If you make these pancakes for your friends, be sure to make extra batter; they'll ask for seconds. Usually pancakes do not provide "long burning fuel," but these do. Serve them with pure maple syrup.

Mix the dry ingredients together in a bowl.

In a separate large bowl, whisk the egg with the milk. Mix the dry ingredients into the milk and stir in the rice.

Heat 1 teaspoon butter or oil in a heavy skillet. When the skillet is hot and the butter sizzles, ladle a large spoonful of batter into it. When air bubbles appear on the top, flip the pancakes and cook for a minute until brown. Remove from the skillet and keep warm in the oven until all are made.

1 cup whole wheat pastry flour

¹/₂ teaspoon salt

¹/₂ teaspoon baking soda

1 egg

1 cup milk (or vanilla soy milk)

¹/₂ cup cooked brown rice

Butter or oil for frying

SERVES 4

Buckwheat Pancakes

½ cup buckwheat flour

½ cup whole wheat pastry flour

½ teaspoon salt

½ teaspoon baking powder

I egg

I cup milk (or plain soy milk)

I tablespoon canola oil

Butter or oil for frying

SERVES 4

Buckwheat pancakes have a wonderful nutty flavor. Top them with pure maple syrup or yogurt and fruit.

Sift together the dry ingredients.

In a large bowl, whisk together the egg, milk, and oil. Stir the dry ingredients into the milk and mix well.

Heat 1 teaspoon of butter or oil in a large skillet. When the skillet is hot and the butter sizzles, ladle a large spoonful of batter into it. When air bubbles appear on the top, flip the pancakes and cook for a minute until brown. Remove from the skillet and keep warm in the oven until all are made.

Spoon Bread

Spoon bread is one of my favorite breakfasts. When I was a child, my mother used to make it for special occasions. I bake it in a round, shallow ceramic baking dish and serve it with maple syrup or butter and salt and pepper. It's essentially a cornmeal soufflé and should be served as soon as it comes out of the oven.

Preheat the oven to 400 degrees.

Mix the cornmeal and baking powder together. In a medium-size saucepan, bring the water and salt to a full boil. Slowly whisk in the cornmeal. Add the milk and cook over medium heat for 10 minutes. Stir in the butter.

Separate the eggs. Beat the whites until stiff. Remove the cornmeal from the stove and whisk in the egg yolks. Fold in the whites and pour the mixture into a buttered 2-quart casserole dish.

Place in the middle rack of the oven and turn down the temperature to 375 degrees. Bake for 30 minutes. To make sure it is well cooked, plunge a thin knife into the center and if it comes out clean, the soufflé is done. Be careful when you open and close the door of the oven; too much of a jolt will cause the soufflé to fall. Serve immediately.

1 cup yellow cornmeal

1 teaspoon baking powder

1 ½ cups boiling water

¼ teaspoon salt

1 cup milk (or plain soy milk)

4 tablespoons butter

3 eggs

SERVES 4

Breakfast Crepes

½ cup buckwheat flour

½ cup whole wheat pastry flour

½ teaspoon salt

½ teaspoon baking powder

1 egg

1 tablespoon canola oil

1 ½ to 2 cups milk

Butter for frying

14 6-INCH CREPES

For breakfast, fill these crepes with unsweetened jams or Hot Stewed Fruits with Ricotta (page 184). Buckwheat has a tendency to absorb liquid, so while the batter might start out thin enough, you may need to add more milk as you go along. You can make crepes in advance and freeze them. Defrost in the refrigerator the night before you plan to serve them.

Sift together the dry ingredients. In a large bowl, whisk together the egg, oil, and 1 ½ cups milk. Combine with the dry ingredients and mix well. The batter should be quite thin, with a ribbonlike consistency when you pour it from a spoon. It may become thicker as it sits, so add more milk.

The most important tool for making crepes is the crepe pan. It should be well seasoned. Over medium heat, add a tiny amount of butter to a 7-inch crepe pan. When the butter sizzles, ladle a large spoonful of batter into the center of the pan. Immediately tilt the pan in a circular motion so the batter covers the surface evenly and moves to all edges. It should be thin. Cook a minute until brown, turn over, cook another minute, and remove by lifting up a corner of the crepe, sliding a spatula underneath, and sliding the crepe out onto a plate. Continue in this manner, every so often adding more butter to the pan, until all the batter is gone. Stack the crepes on top of one another.

Spread the jam or filling in the center of the crepe and roll it. Keep warm in the oven before serving. Top with Yogurt-Orange Sauce (next page) and serve.

To freeze, layer the crepes with wax paper. Cover with plastic wrap and place in the freezer.

YOGURT-ORANGE SAUCE

1 cup plain yogurt

$\frac{1}{2}$ cup fresh orange juice

2 tablespoons honey or maple syrup

Mix the yogurt and orange juice together. Sweeten to taste with honey or maple syrup.

Popovers

1 cup whole wheat pastry flour

½ teaspoon salt

1 cup milk (or vanilla soy milk)

3 eggs

2 tablespoons canola oil

MAKES 12

Popovers are wonderful to serve for breakfast. They are fast and easy to cook, and always a special treat served with homemade jams.

Preheat the oven to 450 degrees.

In a mixing bowl, combine the flour and the salt. In a separate large bowl, mix together the milk, eggs, and oil. Stir in the flour and mix well. Do not beat the batter.

Heat a muffin tin in the oven, then oil it well.

Ladle the hot muffin cups two-thirds full with batter. Bake in the center of the oven for 35 minutes. Serve immediately (they will stay puffed for 5 minutes).

These muffins are quick and fun to make. They taste wonderful, and the smell of them baking is sure to endear you to all around.

This is a basic muffin recipe. For variation, add chopped fresh fruit, nuts, poppy seeds, or dried cranberries. You can make banana walnut muffins, or poppy seed banana muffins, or apple muffins, cranberry muffins, cranberry banana muffins, peach muffins, blueberry muffins, and on and on. If no fresh fruit is available, add a teaspoon of your favorite unsweetened jam as you fill the muffin tin. Fill the muffin cups half full with batter, add a teaspoon of jam, and cover with the rest of the batter.

Preheat the oven to 350 degrees. Sift the dry ingredients together. If making poppy seed muffins, stir in ¼ cup poppy seeds.

In a large mixing bowl, whisk together the eggs, oil, honey, and milk. Stir in the flour. Don't overstir the batter or the muffins will lose their lightness. Stir in chopped fruit or ½ cup nuts.

Ladle the batter into well-oiled muffin tins. Bake in the oven for 30 minutes, or until brown on top.

2 cups whole wheat pastry flour

2 teaspoons baking powder

½ teaspoon salt

2 eggs

¼ cup canola oil

¼ to ½ cup clover honey

1 ½ cups milk (or plain soy milk)

1 cup finely chopped fresh fruit

MAKES 12 SMALL MUFFINS

Scrambled Tofu

3 10-ounce blocks firm tofu

2 tablespoons butter

1 yellow onion, chopped

1 celery rib, minced

1 carrot, minced

1 tablespoon turmeric

1 teaspoon dry mustard

1 tablespoon tamari

Salt

Freshly ground pepper

¼ cup chopped fresh parsley

SERVES 4

Turmeric turns the tofu yellow so it looks like scrambled eggs. We add a few vegetables for flavor, and serve it with pan-fried potatoes and muffins.

At least 1 hour before cooking, rinse the tofu and drain it in a colander. Raise one end of a large cutting board 1 inch off the counter. Place a clean towel on the board and place the tofu on it. Cover the tofu with another clean towel and place a heavy board on top. Press the tofu for 1 hour in this way to remove any excess liquid.

Cut the tofu into cubes. Heat the butter in a large sauté pan. Cook the onion, celery, and carrots over high heat for 3 to 4 minutes, stirring frequently. Add the turmeric and dry mustard. Lower the heat to medium and cook for a couple of minutes. Add the tofu and cook for 20 minutes, stirring frequently. Season with tamari, salt, and freshly ground pepper to taste. Remove from the heat, toss in the fresh parsley, and serve.

Huevos Rancheros

For a hearty breakfast or brunch, serve these Mexican fried eggs with tortillas and Ranchero Sauce.

Heat the oven to 350 degrees and bake the tortillas until crisp. Heat the beans in a saucepan. If you don't have cooked beans on hand, serve the huevos without them. Heat 1 tablespoon of butter or oil in a large skillet that holds 4 eggs at a time. When the butter begins to sizzle, crack the eggs into the pan, one by one, without breaking the yolks. Cover with a lid and cook for 2 minutes, until the whites are set.

Place the crisp tortilla on a plate and cover with a layer of beans. Slide 2 fried eggs onto the beans and cover with Ranchero Sauce. Garnish with a sprinkling of chopped cilantro.

RANCHERO SAUCE

1 tablespoon canola oil
1 cup finely chopped yellow onion
2 medium garlic cloves, minced
1/2 teaspoon dried oregano
1/2 teaspoon chili powder
3 jalapeño chili peppers, seeded and minced
2 cups canned crushed tomatoes
3/4 cup water

MAKES 2 CUPS

4 8-inch whole wheat tortillas
2 cups Black Bean Chili (page 78) or
*   refried beans (page 80)*
8 eggs
Butter or oil for frying eggs
2 cups Ranchero Sauce
Finely chopped fresh cilantro, for
*   garnish*

SERVES 4

Heat the oil in a medium-size saucepan. Add the onions and garlic and cook over high heat for 3 to 4 minutes, stirring frequently. When the onions begin to look translucent, add the oregano and chili powder. Lower the heat and cook for 1 minute. Add the jalapeños, tomatoes, and water. Partially cover with a lid and simmer for 15 minutes.

Hot Stewed Fruits with Ricotta

There is nothing more delicious on a cold winter morning than hot cereal and fruit. One of my favorite breakfasts is a bowl of rice cream with vanilla soy milk and hot stewed fruits on top. The combination makes a wonderful pudding. Packaged rice cream can be bought in natural food stores.

The stewed fruits also make delicious fillings for Breakfast Crepes (page 178).

For dried fruits (apricots, pears, peaches, prunes, and apples): Cut 2 cups of dried fruit into small bite-size pieces. Place them in a large bowl and cover generously with water. Soak overnight.

In a medium saucepan, simmer the fruits in their soaking juice and enough extra water to cover them. Cook over low heat for 30 minutes, partially covered with a lid.

For fresh fruits (apples, strawberries, apricots, and plums): Never peel the fruit. Core and slice into bite-size pieces. Place in a medium saucepan with ½ cup of water. You don't need much water, as the fruits themselves will produce their own juices. Simmer over low heat for 30 minutes, partially covered with a lid. Most fruits don't need sweetening, but add maple syrup or honey to your taste.

As a topping: Mix 1 cup ricotta cheese with 1 cup cottage cheese and serve in a separate bowl along with the stewed fruits. A dollop of ricotta mix on top of hot fruit is wonderful.

Seiko's Sublime Strawberry Rhubarb Sauce

Serve with yogurt for breakfast or with ice cream for late-night TV.

Wash the strawberries and rhubarb. Hull the strawberries with a sharp paring knife and thickly slice them. Place the fruit in a pot with ½ cup of water and simmer until everything is pink, about 20 minutes. Add maple syrup to taste.

1 quart strawberries

10 stalks rhubarb, sliced diagonally ⅓ inch thick

Maple syrup

SERVES 4

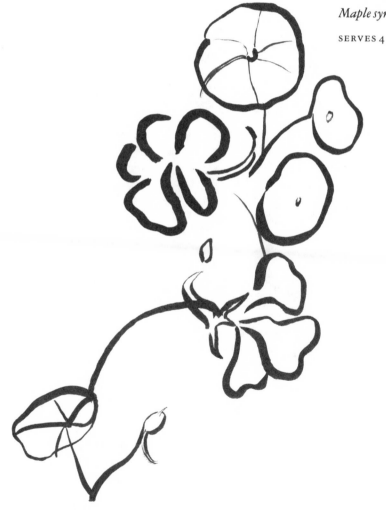

Desserts

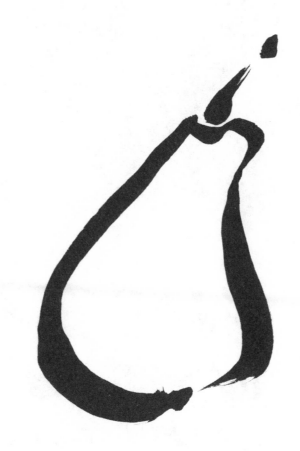

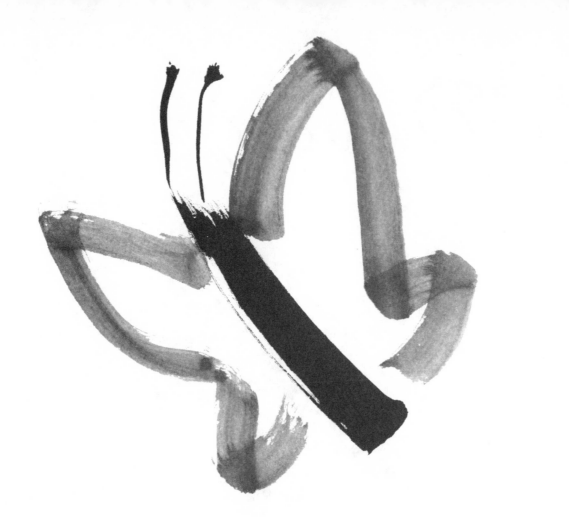

WAKE UP
WAKE UP
BE MY FRIEND
SLEEPING
BUTTERFLY

When you cook with your heart, people can taste it. This is the real secret of great cooking. No fancy techniques are necessary, just the willingness to give yourself wholeheartedly to what you do.

> *"You are the Butterfly—*
> *I the sleeping heart of*
> *Chuang Tzu."*

This poem by Basho refers to the famous story of Chuang Tzu, who dreamt he was a butterfly. When Chuang Tzu awoke he didn't know if he was a butterfly dreaming he was a man or a man dreaming he was a butterfly. The two had merged. Basho wrote this poem when parting from a dear friend to express the profound connection he felt with him.

Have you ever had this experience of there being no separation between you and another person or between you and what you are doing?

As cooks, we can devote ourselves to preparing food that sustains and nurtures our friends and family. We can be one heart, one mind.

Where you are, who you are with, what you are doing, these are not the essentials. What does matter is the spirit that you bring to things. Cutting carrots in the kitchen or conversing with lamas in Tibet is all the same—if your heart is in it.

Desserts

I first learned to cook with Julia Child's wonderful book *Mastering the Art of French Cooking*. It was a magical experience to find that butter, eggs, and chocolate could be transformed into a soufflé or a rich cake. I was so inspired that in the early days of my own restaurant, I would spend hours in the kitchen baking cheesecakes, cream puffs, pies, and chocolate mousses.

The recipes that follow represent my favorite desserts and ones that are more up to date than the heavy creams and chocolates of the past. They are very simple to make and yet elegant. What could be more delicious or beautiful than fruit tarts and pies made in the summer with newly harvested peaches, plums, nectarines, pears, and berries? Fresh fruit ices are refreshing on hot summer days, and in the winter warm custards and bread puddings are wholesome and inviting.

Sweet Tart Pastry

Tarts are fun to make and elegant to serve. The pastry is easy, only taking about ten minutes to prepare. Tart pans have a fluted ring that you can slip off after baking so the pastry stands alone, a sculptured shell filled with beautiful fruits and custards.

In a large bowl, sift together the dry ingredients. Cut the butter into pieces. Using your fingers, crumble the butter into the flour until it is thoroughly mixed and feels like coarse meal. Stir in the water a tiny bit at a time. Add only enough water until the flour forms into a ball. Wrap in wax paper and refrigerate for half an hour.

The trick to making this kind of pastry is not to handle the dough too much. Place the dough onto a lightly floured surface—marble or tile is excellent. Form the dough into a round flat shape and dust the top with flour. With a rolling pin, roll away from you with even strokes to form a circle about ⅛ inch thick. Make sure there is enough flour under the dough to keep it from sticking to the surface. You may need to scatter flour over the rolling pin as well.

When the dough is the size of your tart pan, fold it in half, lay it in the pan, unfold it, and lightly press around the inside edges.

1 ¼ cups whole wheat pastry flour
1 ½ tablespoons sugar
¼ teaspoon salt
½ teaspoon baking powder
6 tablespoons butter
¼ cup ice cold water

MAKES ONE 10-INCH TART

Fruit Tart

1 recipe Sweet Tart Pastry (page 191),
   fitted into a 10-inch tart pan

1/3 cup unsweetened raspberry jam

1/4 cup water

3 large ripe peaches, pitted and sliced
   thin

MAKES ONE 10-INCH TART

For tarts, all you need are the freshest fruits of the season. You can use this same recipe for nectarines, pears, apricots, raspberries, blueberries, apples, and plums. These fruits look beautiful arranged in rosettes and overlapping circles of color and shape. The French are masters of pastry design. I always visit my neighborhood patisserie for inspiration.

Preheat the oven to 375 degrees. Prepare the tart pastry.

In a small saucepan, warm the raspberry jam with water to make a thin glaze. Brush the bottom of the pastry shell with a thin covering of glaze.

Wash the peaches and cut them in half. Remove the pits, cutting in quarters and then in thin slices. Arrange them in the pastry by overlapping the slices in a circle, beginning at the outer edge, working around, and then in toward the center.

Cover lightly with foil and bake for 30 minutes. Uncover and bake another 10 minutes. Remove the tart from the oven. Remove the fluted ring and slide the tart onto a serving plate. Brush a warm glaze of raspberry jam over all the peaches and edges of the crust.

Lemon Tart with Berries

The tanginess of fresh lemon, combined with the delicate sweetness of fresh picked blueberries or raspberries, makes a wonderful, refreshing desert. You can make the lemon cream in advance. It keeps well for three or four days.

Preheat the oven to 375 degrees. Prepare the tart pastry and bake it in the lower third of the oven. After 5 minutes, check it and if any air bubbles have developed, pierce them with a sharp knife. Continue baking for 15 or 20 minutes, until brown. Cool to room temperature before filling with the lemon cream.

In a saucepan, mix together all the lemon cream ingredients except the egg yolks, vanilla, and nutmeg. Cook over medium-low heat, stirring constantly, for 15 minutes. This gives the flour time to cook and the arrowroot time to thicken. Do not bring to a boil.

In a separate bowl, whisk the egg yolks. Slowly whisk ½ cup of the hot cream into the eggs. Then slowly whisk this egg mixture back into the saucepan and continue to stir over medium heat for another 5 to 10 minutes, until the cream becomes quite thick. Do not bring to a boil. Remove from the stove. Stir in the vanilla and nutmeg. Pour into a bowl, cover the surface with plastic wrap to avoid a thick skin forming over the top, and cool in the refrigerator.

Fill the pastry shell with the cooled lemon cream. Arrange the raspberries on top. In a saucepan, heat the raspberry jam over medium-low heat with enough water to make a thin glaze. With a pastry brush, paint a thin coating of glaze over the raspberries and the edges of the tart.

1 recipe Sweet Tart Pastry (page 191)

LEMON CREAM:

½ cup clover honey

⅓ cup unbleached white flour

3 tablespoons arrowroot powder

⅓ cup lemon juice

1¼ cups water

4 egg yolks

1 teaspoon vanilla extract

Pinch of grated nutmeg

1 pint fresh raspberries

½ cup unsweetened raspberry jam

MAKES ONE 10-INCH TART

Pear Custard Tart

1 recipe Pastry Dough (page 195)

6 medium-large ripe pears

2 cups milk or unsweetened soy milk

¼ cup clover honey

2 eggs

Pinch of grated nutmeg

Pinch of ground cinnamon

1 teaspoon pure vanilla extract

MAKES ONE 10 × 14-INCH COOKIE

SHEET–SIZE TART

Bake this tart on a square cookie sheet or square tart pan, and arrange the pear slices in overlapping rectangular rows. Use any fresh fruit in season: apples, pears, apricots, nectarines, or peaches.

Prepare the pastry dough. Divide it in two. Roll out one-half to fit the upper half of the cookie sheet. Roll out the second half to fit the other half of the cookie sheet. Use your hands to pinch the center together. Scallop the edges to 1 inch high.

Preheat the oven to 375 degrees.

Core the pears and cut into thin slices. Starting at the top of the pastry, place the pears horizontally across and then down in overlapping layers.

Heat the milk and honey in a saucepan over medium heat. In a medium bowl, mix the eggs. Slowly whisk a small amount of hot milk into the eggs and whisk the eggs back into the saucepan of milk. Stir in the spices and vanilla. Remove from the heat and pour over the pears. Place in the oven and bake for 1 hour, until the custard has set.

Pastry Dough

Making pies is easy, and the more you do it, the more it becomes like second nature. Whenever I make a pie I feel like a sculptor. I form a shape around the fruit with the pastry. I make designs on the top with a fork and paint it with an egg glaze. I mold the sides into scallop shapes and sometimes make a crisscross lattice design across the top.

Preheat the oven to 350 degrees.

In a large bowl, sift together the flour, salt, and sugar (if using). Cut the butter into pieces. Using your fingers, crumble the butter into the flour until it is thoroughly mixed and feels like coarse meal. Stir in the water a tiny bit at a time. Add only enough water until the flour forms into a ball. Wrap in wax paper and refrigerate for half an hour.

Cut the dough in half. Dust some flour onto your rolling surface and onto your rolling pin. Form the dough into a round flat shape, dust the top with flour, and roll away from you with even strokes. Roll into a circle ¼ inch thick and about 2 inches larger than your pie plate. Move the dough around to make sure it is not sticking to the table surface. If it starts to stick, dust some flour underneath. Fold the dough in half, lay it in the pie plate, and unfold.

Put your filling into the pie and then roll out the top half of the crust. Fold the dough in half and lay this top layer over your filling. Unfold it. Trim the edges by running a small knife around the rim of the pie plate.

With the first 2 fingers of your right hand, pinch the edges of the dough around your left thumb. This will give the pie beautiful scalloped edges. With a fork, prick a design on the top. Beat the egg yolk and lightly brush it over the top of the crust. Bake for 30 to 40 minutes, until the crust is brown. Let it cool for 10 minutes before serving.

2 cups whole wheat pastry flour

¼ teaspoon salt

1 teaspoon sugar (optional)

12 tablespoons (1½ sticks) butter

¼ to ½ cup ice cold water

1 egg yolk

MAKES ONE 9-INCH DEEP-DISH PIE

Deep-Dish Apple Pie

3 pounds Granny Smith, Jonathan, or
    Baldwin apples

1 teaspoon ground cinnamon

1 tablespoon pure vanilla extract

2 tablespoons arrowroot powder

1 recipe Pastry Dough (page 195)

1 egg yolk

MAKES ONE 9-INCH PIE

When I was baking for The Beat'n Path Cafe, I made a deep-dish apple pie every day. I would pile the apples four or five inches high. During the baking, the apples would condense in size, but the crust would remain floating high in the air. It was most impressive looking, and when you cut into it the flaky crust fell down around the apples like clouds.

When I make apple or peach pies, I rarely add sweetener. I love the fruit flavors as they are. If you really want to sweeten a pie, mix some candied ginger in with the fruit.

Preheat the oven to 350 degrees.

Don't peel the apples. Core and slice them into ½-inch bite-size pieces. In a large bowl, toss them with the cinnamon, vanilla, and arrowroot.

Roll out the bottom of the pastry dough and place in a pie plate. Spoon the apples into the pastry. Roll out the top crust. Fold in half and unfold on top of the apples. Run a small knife around the edge of the pie plate, cutting off any extra dough. Using the first 2 fingers of your right hand, pinch the edges of the dough around your left thumb to scallop the edges.

Lightly beat the egg yolk with a tablespoon of water and brush it over the crust. With a fork or a small knife, prick a design on the top. This will keep the crust from cracking open during baking. Bake for 45 minutes, until the crust is golden brown. Cool for 10 minutes before serving.

Linzertorte

This is one of my favorite pastries to make. It is traditionally made with almonds and raspberry preserves, but recently I substituted walnuts for the almonds and it was delicious. It's festive looking with the red raspberries peeking out through the lattice crust.

Preheat the oven to 325 degrees.

In a large bowl, cream the butter and honey. Stir in the lemon zest and eggs.

In another bowl, sift the nuts with the flour, spices, salt, and baking powder. Pour into the bowl with the butter and honey and mix well.

Butter or oil a 10-inch tart pan. Evenly spread three-quarters of the batter into it. Brush a ⅛-inch layer of raspberry preserves over the top. Place the remaining dough in a pastry bag. Squeeze a ring of pastry around the edge of the tart pan and make a lattice pattern on the top.

Bake for 45 to 50 minutes, until the pastry is golden brown and the preserves are bubbling. Serve either warm or cool.

½ pound (2 sticks) butter

¾ cup clover honey

2 teaspoons grated lemon zest

2 eggs

1¼ cups finely ground almonds or walnuts

1¾ cups whole wheat pastry flour

½ teaspoon ground cinnamon

¼ teaspoon ground cloves

¼ teaspoon salt

1 teaspoon baking powder

⅔ cup unsweetened raspberry preserves

MAKES ONE 10-INCH TART

Plum Torte

5 ripe plums

1/2 teaspoon ground cinnamon

1/2 teaspoon grated nutmeg

6 tablespoons butter

1/2 cup clover honey

2 eggs

1 cup whole wheat pastry flour

1 teaspoon baking powder

Pinch of salt

Whipped cream (optional)

Confectioners' sugar (optional)

MAKES ONE 9-INCH TORTE

This torte is a combination cake and fruit tart. The batter will rise a little and the fruit will cook into the cake. Besides plums, you can use any seasonal fresh fruit: apples, peaches, berries, and pears. They will all be delicious. Make this torte in a 9-inch springform pan.

Preheat the oven to 350 degrees.

Cut the plums in half. Remove the pits and cut into 1/4-inch-thick slices. Combine them in a bowl with the cinnamon and nutmeg. Set aside.

In a large bowl, cream the butter with the honey, then stir in the eggs. In a separate bowl, sift all the dry ingredients together. Combine with the creamed butter.

Oil the bottom and sides of the springform pan. Spread the batter evenly over the bottom. Place the sliced plums, skin side up, on top of the batter, pressing down lightly. Arrange the fruit in a circular pattern.

Bake in the oven for 45 to 60 minutes, until the cake is golden brown and firm. Serve with whipped cream or dusted with confectioners' sugar.

Fresh Fruit Ices

Colorful ices make wonderfully refreshing desserts. They are easy to make and can be made with any fresh fruit in season or with unsweetened fruit juice. Use the basic recipes below for tangerines, oranges, mangoes, pineapples, raspberries, strawberries, grapes, and apricots. Most of the ices don't need sweetener, unless it's a tart lemon or lime.

Pineapple Lime Ice

In a food processor, blend all the ingredients together. Strain the blended liquid, discarding any pulp from the pineapple, and pour the thick juice into a bowl. Place in the freezer. After 2 or 3 hours, remove from the freezer and break the ice into large chunks. Blend again in the food processor until smooth and creamy. Return to the freezer for at least 30 more minutes until serving.

To serve, scoop the ice onto serving plates or into sherbert glasses. Garnish with sprigs of fresh mint or slices of lime.

2 cups chopped fresh pineapple

6 tablespoons lime juice

2 tablespoons honey

2 tablespoons grated lime zest

¹/₂ cup water

Sprigs of fresh mint or lime slices, for garnish

SERVES 4

Lemon Ice

Combine all ingredients in a food processor and blend until smooth. Pour into a bowl and freeze for 2 to 3 hours. Break the frozen ice into large chunks and blend again in the food processor until smooth and creamy. Return to the freezer for at least 30 more minutes until serving. Scoop the ice into sherbert glasses and garnish with fresh mint.

²/₃ cup lemon juice

3 cups water

1 cup clover honey

Fresh mint, for garnish

SERVES 4

Raspberry Ice

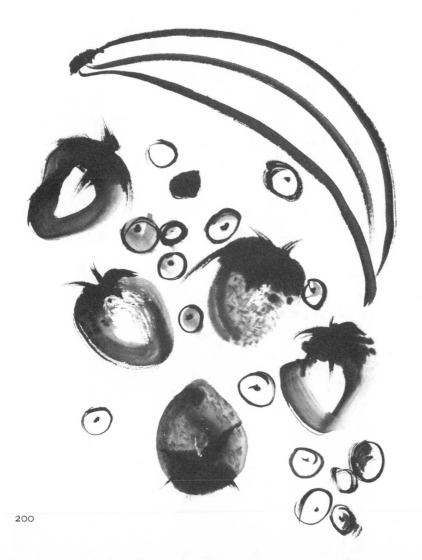

16 ounces unsweetened raspberry juice

SERVES 4 TO 6

Many stores carry a wide variety of unsweetened fruit juices that are perfect for making ices.

Pour the juice into a bowl and place in the freezer for 2 to 3 hours. Break the frozen juice into large chunks and blend in a food processor until smooth and creamy. Return to the freezer for at least another 30 minutes until serving. Scoop the ice into sherbert glasses and serve with your favorite cookies.

Apple Pudding

This pudding is one of the easiest and most delicious desserts I have ever come across, and one of the only recipes I have carried over from my macrobiotic days. It is made primarily with apple juice and agar-agar, a seaweed sometimes called Kanten. The agar has no taste; it acts like gelatin. You can buy it in most natural food stores, where it comes in flakes or bars.

Place the apple juice in a large saucepan. Break the bar of agar-agar into pieces, add it to the apple juice, and cook over medium-high heat, stirring to mix the agar-agar as it dissolves. When the juice begins to boil, immediately reduce the heat and simmer for 15 minutes.

Pour the juice into a flat pan and allow it to cool until it becomes firm, about 1 hour. To speed up the process, you can put it in the refrigerator or freezer.

In a food processor, blend the firm apple juice with the tahini and vanilla until it becomes smooth like a custard. Chill in the refrigerator for 1 hour. Serve in sherbert glasses and top with fresh strawberries.

4 cups unsweetened apple juice

.5-ounce package of agar-agar in bars

4 tablespoons tahini

1 ½ tablespoons pure vanilla extract

Fresh strawberries for topping

SERVES 4

Ginger Custard with Lime

1 tablespoon juice from grated fresh
  ginger
2 1/2 cups milk or plain soy milk
1/2 cup pure maple syrup
2 eggs
3 egg yolks
1/2 teaspoon pure vanilla extract

SERVES 4 TO 6

This is a refreshing custard flavored with ginger and served with slices of lime. We make it with nonfat milk or unflavored soy milk, and it is much lighter than the traditional flan or caramel custard. Make it in individual custard cups or in one large baking dish. Garnish it with slivers of candied ginger and a sprig of mint.

Preheat the oven to 325 degrees.

Peel and finely grate 2 inches of ginger. Squeeze it with your hands or in a towel, so that you extract 1 tablespoon of juice. Set it aside.

In a large saucepan, bring the milk and maple syrup to just below simmering. Remove from the heat and stir in the ginger juice.

In a mixing bowl, whisk all the eggs; slowly whisk in some of the hot milk. When the eggs and milk are well mixed, pour back into the saucepan and return to the stove. Over medium heat, bring the custard to just below simmer, stirring frequently. Remove from the stove and stir in the vanilla.

Pour the custard into individual custard cups or a large baking dish. Set the custards in a pan that is deep enough to pour hot water halfway up the sides of the custard dishes. Bake in the oven for 1 hour. If you make this custard with soy milk, it will take longer to bake. When the custard is firm and a knife inserted comes out clean, remove from the oven. Cool and serve with slices of lime.

Crème Anglaise

This is a luscious and creamy sauce. Serve it over fresh-picked berries, peaches, and nectarines. It makes a wonderful topping for fruit crisps.

In a medium bowl, beat the egg yolks.

In a saucepan, heat the milk and honey together. When the honey has thoroughly dissolved and the milk is quite hot, whisk half the milk into the eggs. Then slowly whisk this mixture back into the saucepan of milk. Continue to cook over medium heat, stirring constantly. As it cooks it will thicken slightly. Do not bring it to a boil or it will curdle.

When your spoon becomes thickly coated with the custard, it is done. Immediately remove from the heat and stir in the cinnamon and vanilla. Cool before serving.

4 egg yolks

2 cups milk

1/2 cup clover honey

1/2 teaspoon ground cinnamon

1 tablespoon pure vanilla extract

MAKES 2 CUPS

Maple Bread Pudding

1 quart lowfat milk (or vanilla soy
   milk)

4 eggs

1 1/2 teaspoons vanilla extract

1/4 cup dark rum

1/2 cup pure maple syrup

4 cups dry whole wheat bread, cut in
   cubes

2 ripe pears

3/4 cup raisins

3/4 cup chopped walnuts

SERVES 4 TO 6

What better use for odds and ends of bread than old-fashioned bread pudding. For this recipe, use whole wheat bread and pure maple syrup. Serve with whipped cream flavored with a touch of vanilla and honey.

Preheat the oven to 350 degrees.

In a large mixing bowl, whisk the milk with the eggs, vanilla, rum, and maple syrup. Stir in the bread. Let sit for 10 minutes.

In the meantime, peel and core the pears. Slice into small bite-size pieces. Butter a 2-quart casserole dish. Stir the pears, raisins, and walnuts into the soaked bread. Mix well and pour into the casserole dish.

Bake in the oven for 1 hour, or until the pudding has set well and is brown on top. Serve with whipped cream.

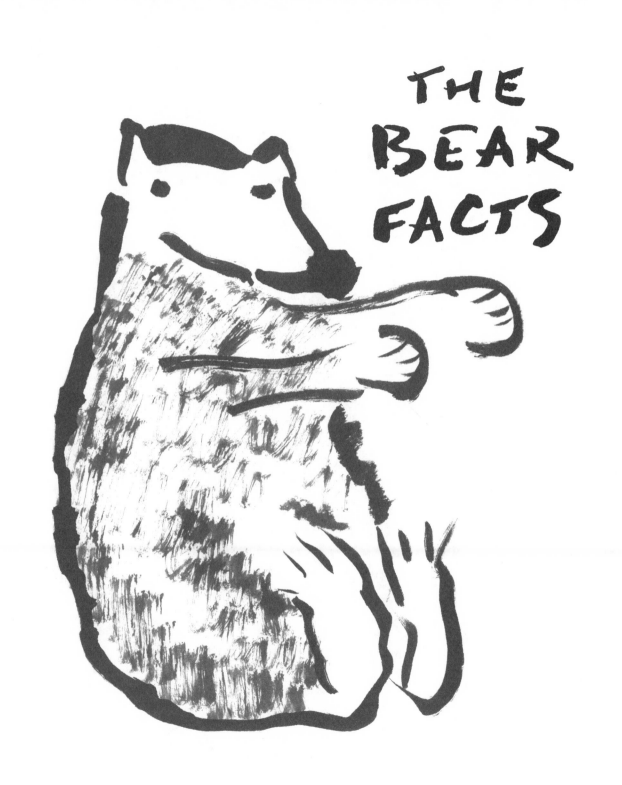

THE BEAR FACTS

Menus

Here are some menu ideas that have been created for all sorts of occasions, from a simple quick lunch to more formal gatherings. Each meal has been planned with tastes, colors, textures, and nutritional balance in mind.

When planning a menu, I like to include a combination of grains and beans or tofu, with fresh vegetables and greens. The grains and beans together make up a complete protein. The vegetables and greens provide carbohydrates, vitamins, and minerals for a well-balanced diet.

It's not hard to create meals that are balanced as well as delicious and elegant to serve. Here are a few examples for an evening dinner: Black Bean Chili served with tortillas or corn bread, accompanied by Jicama and Avocado Salad. Or Mushroom Stroganoff with Baked Tomatoes and a mixed green salad. Sounds appetizing, doesn't it?

If your meal is simple, with just a soup and salad, toss a few cooked beans into the salad and accompany it with whole wheat bruschetta. Serve a selection of two or three salads with the Vietnamese Spring Rolls and Asian-Style Peanut Sauce. Make an elegant dinner with curried couscous pilaf, roasted vegetables, and a peach tart for dessert.

When I eat lightly with fresh vegetable greens, fruits, and whole grains, I don't have to eat a great deal to be satisfied. And what could be more satisfying than fresh corn picked just that morning, with a salad of summer tomatoes and steamed broccoli, or an asparagus risotto flavored delicately with white wine, and a raspberry lemon tart for dessert?

For Luncheon Parties:

Corn Chowder
Tostadas with Tomato Salsa, Avocado, and Black Olives
Jicama with Lime

Miso Soup
Cold Soba Noodles topped with East West Salsa
Platters of cucumber sushi

Spicy Pea Soup
Quesadillas
Roasted Autumn Vegetables
Linzertorte

Szechuan Green Beans and Soba
Thai Carrot Salad with Peanuts
Ginger Custard with Lime

Summer Garden Pizza
Mesclun Salad with Orange Raspberry Vinaigrette
Lemon Tart with Berries

For Special Dinners:

Pesto Pizza
Avocado and Red Peppers
Corn on the cob
Fresh strawberries with Crème Anglaise

Coconut Curry Vegetables served on top of brown rice
Summer Mint and Apple Chutney
Green salad with Ewa's Honey Mustard Dressing

Mushroom Stroganoff
Baked Tomatoes
Mesclun Salad
Fresh fruit

Mushroom Enchiladas with Red Pepper Sauce
Green salad with Chili Lime Basil Dressing
Lemon Ice with mint

Spicy Squash Stew
Basmati rice
Assortment of chutneys
Yogurt Raita with Cucumber
Roasted cashew nuts
Apple Pudding

Carrot Soup
Swiss Chard and Tomato Tart
Mesclun Salad
Raspberry Ice

For Barbecues and Summer Lunches:

Hot and Spicy Cajun Shish Kebabs served with rice
Corn on the cob
Cajun Coleslaw
Plum Torte

Southwestern Potato Pancakes with Cilantro Pesto
Baked Tomatoes
Deep-Dish Apple Pie

Grilled Polenta with Pesto
Marinated Tomatoes
Potato Salad

For Summer Dinners:

Rigatoni with Japanese Eggplants and Basil
Zucchini Salad
Fresh fruit

Summer Vegetable Soup with Basil Sauce
Asparagus Risotto
Mesclun Salad
Pear Custard Tart

Cold Soba Noodles with Orange Raspberry Vinaigrette
Pear, Jicama, and Beet Salad
Ginger Custard with Lime

For Dinners:

Black Bean Soup
Tostadas with Red Pepper Sauce and Melted Cheese
Cajun Coleslaw

Mediterranean Green Salad
Roasted Autumn Vegetables
Bruschetta with Tomatoes and Basil
Linzertorte

Lentil Soup with Mint
Broccoli, Shiitake, and Tomato Salad
Wild Rice Pilaf
Maple Bread Pudding

Refried Bean Burrito with Salsa Verde
Jicama and Avocado Salad
Deep-Dish Apple Pie

Cauliflower Gratin
Red Rice Pilaf
Broccoli Salad with Tofu and Chili Lime Basil Dressing
Lemon Ice

Zucchini Fritters topped with Béchamel Sauce
Mesclun Salad
Fresh peaches with Crème Anglaise

BITTER TEA SWEETENED WITH 2 LUMPS

Glossary of Ingredients

Aduki Beans: These sweet and flavorful small dry red beans are grown in Japan and the United States. They are quick to cook and the easiest of all beans to digest. They make delicious soups and stews, and are wonderful in salads. In Japan they are made into sweets.

Agar-agar or Kanten: Agar-agar is a sea vegetable that acts just like gelatin. It contains many minerals and vitamins. You can buy it in powder, flakes, or bars. In natural food stores it is expensive, but in Japanese markets it costs considerably less. It's a welcome alternative to commercial gelatin.

Arrowroot: This white, starchlike powder is naturally processed from the arrowroot plant, which grows abundantly in the United States. It is a high-quality thickening agent, excellent to use in pies and for thickening sauces.

Balsamic Vinegar: This vinegar is specially aged in wood and made only in Modena, Italy. It has a full-bodied and slightly sweet flavor.

Chilis: Chili peppers have been around for a long time. They have been traced to the Incan and Aztec cultures of 5000 B.C. The heat of chili peppers is measured by an international standard that uses a rating scale of 1 to 120. The jalapeño pepper, which we consider hot, is rated only 15!

Cayenne are dried and crushed into red pepper flakes or ground into a fine red powder. The powder is very hot, and a tiny pinch will often be enough. Cayenne is one of nature's true stimulants. It's good for the heart, improves circulation, and is high in vitamin C. *Dried red pepper flakes* are also very *very* hot. Use them sparingly.

Fresh chili peppers are readily available in most markets. They are related to bell peppers, and have a diversity of flavors. They vary in hotness, depending on growing conditions. When using these chilis, be sure to always remove the seeds and the veins.

Poblano chilis, also called ancho when dried, have a mellow aromatic flavor. They are 3 to 4 inches long, dark green in color, heart-shaped, and relatively mild. *Anaheim chilis* are long and skinny and paler in color than the poblano. Anaheims are mild, rich in flavor, and delicious with corn, green beans, and squash. They are traditionally used for the Mexican dish Chilis Rellenos.

Jalapeño and serrano chilis are *very* hot. They are very small chilis, about two inches long and half an inch wide. They are excellent to use for spicy dishes such as black bean chili or for making hot fiery salsas.

Cilantro: Cilantro (also known as fresh coriander and Chinese parsley) is an herb widely used in Mexican and Asian cooking. It looks like flat-leaf parsley, but has a strong and pungent flavor. Coriander are the seeds of the cilantro plant. They have a sweet nutmeglike flavor and are delicious in curries.

Curry Powder: Curry is a combination of dried and ground spices based on the traditional Indian spice mixture called garam masala. Depending on the taste of the cook, different combinations of spices are used, and there are many to choose from: ginger, basil, mint, lemon grass, black pepper, mustard seeds, turmeric, cayenne, cardamom, nutmeg, cumin, coriander, fenugreek, fennel seeds, chili peppers, saffron, and cinnamon. Commercial curry powder is milder than homemade.

Ginger: Use fresh ginger for its wonderful hot and tangy flavor. It's a good ingredient in dressings and marinades, it spices up stews, flavors custards and flans, and gives a special lift to soups. Keep it refrigerated. Ground ginger is not a substitute for fresh ginger.

Ginger is a natural stimulant, excellent for circulation and good for colds. It helps the body recover from stress and fatigue.

Honey: Honey is a complex carbohydrate that contains minerals, vitamins, and enzymes. Clover honey has a delicate and fragrant taste, and is good to use in cooking and baking.

Jicama: Jicama is a delicious and refreshing Mexican root vegetable. Brown on the outside, but pure white, crisp, and sweet on the inside, it's great in salads and wonderful when combined with fresh fruits and a touch of cayenne.

Kombu: Kombu is a wide, thick, dark green seaweed that grows in the ocean. Dried, it is a staple of Japanese cooking and is used for making Dashi broth and other soup stock. It's recently been discovered that drinking kombu broth lowers blood pressure and improves the condition of the heart.

Lovage: I use lovage constantly in my cooking. It looks like a cross between celery leaves and large Italian parsley and has a fresh strong celery taste. It's great in soups, minced in tofu salads and rice dishes, and it goes very well with tomatoes. It's not readily found in the markets but is easy to grow in your garden or window box.

Mirin: Mirin is a sweet cooking wine, a staple in Japanese cuisine.

Miso: Miso is a paste made of fermented soybeans and sea salt. It is rich in protein and comes in different varieties and strengths, depending on the length of fermentation. The sweetest and lightest tasting is the pale yellow Saigyo miso. Red miso has a strong intense flavor. Use miso paste in soups, sauces, and dressings.

Noodles: *Soba* and *Udon* noodles are among Japan's most popular foods. There are restaurants devoted solely to serving these noodles. Sobas are made from buckwheat flour and have a delicious, toasted flavor. I buy them in Japanese markets where they are much less expensive than in natural food stores. Udon noodles are wide flat noodles made from wheat flour.

Nori: The Japanese eat 9 billion sheets of nori a year. It's a sea vegetable that is dried into thin square sheets measuring seven by eight inches. It's roasted over a flame until it becomes green and looks like exotic handmade paper. It is used to make sushi and can also be roasted and cut into strips for very tasty condiments and garnishes.

Oils: The best oils to use are cold-pressed *monounsaturated oils* such as canola oil and extra virgin olive oil. It's been proven that such oils do *not* increase the risk of cardiovascular disease.

Olive oil has been used for centuries in the Mediterranean. Extra virgin olive oil comes from the first pressing of the olives. It is fragrant and flavorful and best used in salad dressings. Virgin olive oil comes from the second pressing of the olives and is used for most cooking. Canola oil is a traditional oil of India and southern China. It has very little flavor and is good to use in stir-fries and for cooking chilis and stews.

Unsaturated oils, like safflower, walnut, and sunflower seed, are unstable oils that have a tendency to turn rancid easily. If you use these oils, keep them refrigerated.

Parmesan Cheese: This is a hard, grating cheese. The best kind is Parmegiana Reggiano, which has a buttery and nutty flavor. Buy it by the piece and grate it fresh as needed. Wrap it tightly and keep it refrigerated.

Rice: Brown rice comes in three varieties; short-, medium-, and long-grain. Long-grain rice is elegant to serve; short-grain is chewy with a sweet taste.

Basmati rice was originally grown in the foothills of the Himalayas. It is named for the Basmati flower that blooms only in India. The rice has a delicate perfumed flavor that is lovely in risottos, or served with steamed vegetables.

Arborio rice is grown in Italy. It is perfect for making risottos because of its creamy consistency when cooked. Although expensive, it is well worth it.

Rice Vinegar: A tart vinegar made from rice, it is a staple of Japanese cooking.

Sake: Sake is a sweet-tasting rice wine that is widely used in Japanese cooking. It contains about 15 percent alcohol. It tenderizes and enhances the flavor of foods.

Shiitake Mushrooms: Many supermarkets now carry fresh shiitake mushrooms. The dried variety is available in Japanese markets and natural food stores. They have a rich, earthy flavor like wild mushrooms. Always discard the stems of these mushrooms or save them for use in soup stocks.

Shiitakes are Japan's most popular mushroom. They have many medicinal qualities and are reputed to be helpful in preventing high blood pressure and cancer.

Soy Milk: Soy milk is an excellent substitute for regular milk. It is high in protein and contains less fat than regular milk. It's made from soybeans that have been simmered in water, then pressed through a sieve. The milk is commercially available either plain or sweetened with honey or barley malt.

For baking or for making sauces, use unsweetened soy milk. Many of the sweetened varieties have a tan color, which is unsuitable for custards, lemon creams, and white sauces.

Tahini: A smooth, creamy butter made from sesame seeds, it is rich in calcium and protein.

Tamari: Tamari, a fermented soybean product, has a rich taste. I use it instead of salt to deepen the flavors of my cooking. It is an excellent substitute for salt: 1 tablespoon tamari = ½ teaspoon salt.

Tofu: Tofu is a staple of both vegetarian and Asian cooking. It is a wonder food made from soybeans. The beans are cooked, then blended with water and mixed with a natural solidifier. The resulting "curds" are then pressed into small cakes. These cakes ar either firm or soft. The firm style is great for sautés, in salads, and grilled. The soft variety is perfect for salad dressings and tofu creams used in lasagnes and vegetable tarts.

Tofu itself has very little taste, but it has a tremendous ability to absorb flavors. It is rich in protein and minerals and low in cholesterol. Buy tofu that contains no chemical preservatives. Supermarkets carry an assortment of tofu and health food stores sell the best quality. Keep it refrigerated, covered with water, for up to one week.

Tomatillos: These vegetables are sometimes called Mexican green tomatoes. They are covered in a pale green paper husk and have a fresh, lemony taste. You can find them in Mexican markets and supermarkets carrying a large variety of Mexican food.

Tortillas and Tacos: A staple food of Mexico, tortillas are thin, flat unleavened breads that vary in diameter from six inches to twelve or fourteen inches. They are folded around beans and cheese, or crisped into tortilla chips and eaten with guacamole and salsas. Fried tortillas become taco shells that are filled with lettuce, tomatoes, and other ingredients. They are made from corn or wheat flour. Tortillas from the southwestern United States are made from blue cornmeal.

Wasabi: Wasabi is a Japanese powdered horseradish made from the root of the wasabi plant. This green, hot, spicy powder is served with Japanese sushi. It is mixed with a small amount of water to make a thick paste. It does not keep, so only make as much as you need.

What Is Zen: A Brief Explanation

by Eido Tai Shimano Roshi, Abbot of The Zen Studies Society

A special transmission outside the scriptures;
No dependence on words and letters;
Direct pointing to the mind of man;
Seeing into one's nature and attaining Buddhahood.

BODHIDHARMA

The special transmission of Zen is the realization of the Buddha's enlightenment itself, in one's own life, in one's own time. This experience has been realized by Zen students and confirmed by their teachers for over 2500 years.

Central and indispensable to Zen is daily Zazen practice. It is this practice that is the "direct pointing to the mind of man." Zazen melts away the mind-forged distances that separate man from himself, leads one beyond himself as knower, to himself as known. In Zazen, there is no reality outside what exists here and now. Each moment, each act is inherently Buddha nature. While sorrow and joy, anxiety and imperturbability cannot be avoided, by not clinging to them we find ourselves free of them, no longer pulled this way and that. With this self-mastery comes composure and tranquility of mind, but these are by-products of Zazen rather than its goals.

Zazen is a Japanese term consisting of two characters: *za*, "to sit (cross-legged)," and *zen*, from the Sanskrit *dhyana*, meaning at once "concentration, dynamic stillness, and contemplation." The means toward the realization of one's original nature as well as the realization itself, Zazen is both something one does—sitting cross-legged, with proper posture and correct breathing—and something one essentially is. To emphasize one aspect at the expense of the other is to misunderstand this subtle and profound practice.

In ordinary experience, being and doing are separated: What one does is cut off from what one is, and conversely. Such separation leads inevitably to the condition of self-alienation. Particularly in this century, this condition has become acute. With time and sincere effort in Zazen practice, mind and body, inside and outside, self and other are experienced as one. This condition of effortless concentration is known as Samadhi.

In the clarity of Samadhi-liveliness, dissatisfaction and the sense of the meaninglessness of modern life vanish. No longer searching for answers externally, the student journeys within to reach the moving spirit of the Buddha—his own Self-Nature.

Through devotion and persistence, the aims of Zazen practice are eventually realized. The first is Enlightenment. With this experience, Samadhi is fulfilled; mind and body, the self and the universe are seen to have been one reality from the beginning. The second and more difficult aim is the actualization of the Bodhisattva (Enlightened Being) ideal. This spirit of love and compassion for all beings is developed through continual spiritual purification, the cultivation of a deep sense of responsibility, and, most importantly, self-discipline. As one's practice ripens, one becomes more alive, more creative, filled with the longing to actualize the Bodhisattva spirit in every moment and every aspect of daily life.

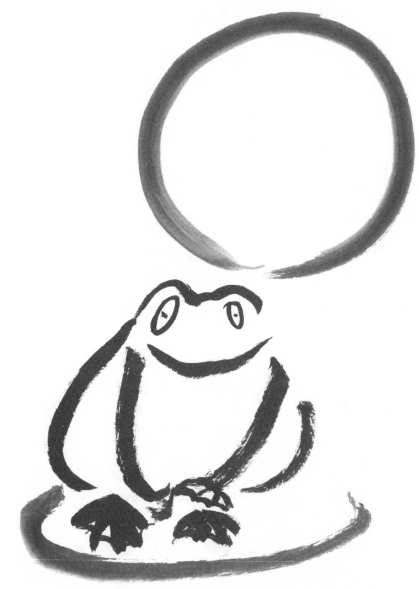

Sensory Awareness:
"The Rediscovery of Experiencing"

by Kenneth McCarthy

In an era when public relations is often a substitute for substance, and the human potential movement seems at times like a 24-hour convenience store, it's worthwhile taking a fresh look at the roots of the movement and reminding ourselves of its profound and revolutionary origins. Some of the pioneers are no longer with us. But Charlotte Selver, a teacher of teachers and a touchstone of dedication and integrity, is still offering her unique and innovative work.

In 1938, almost 50 years ago, Selver came to the United States from Germany, bringing a practice that continues to have an enormous influence on the way we define ourselves as human beings. The intention of this practice is simply to create an opportunity for the individual to experience the unity of mind and body. In the world of the '30s and '40s, this was a strange idea in most circles. The separateness and superiority of the intellect was a concept so firmly ingrained that to question it seemed absurd. The body was something to ignore, transcend, or improve through exercise.

Within this intellectual climate, Selver worked indomitably to establish an appreciation of "entire being," the context within which all the potentials of the human being can continue to unfold.

In 1963, Selver offered the first workshops in nonverbal experimentation at Esalen Institute. Many who went on to make names for themselves in various forms of "awareness training" attended those early seminars. Indeed, Selver coined the term "sensory awareness," now often used so carelessly, in 1950 to describe her work. And Selver has had a profound impact on humanistic psychology, in part due to her influence on some of the major theorists and writers of this century.

For example, in the 1940s, Erich Fromm introduced Selver at the New School for Social Research in New York, where she presented the first courses in "body awareness" given at that institution.

Fritz Perls spent a year and a half studying with her and incorporated many of her ideas into his Gestalt therapy. In particular, he took from her his emphasis on awareness and on being, rather than having, an organism.

Alan Watts, who gave joint seminars with Selver before her move to California, called her work "living Zen." The West Coast Zen community enthusiastically embraced sensory awareness and saw it as very much in the spirit of their own pursuits. Shunryu Suzuki Roshi, who collaborated with Selver in a benefit workshop for his Tassajara Zen monastery, called their practice "the inner experience of entire being, the pure flow of sensory awareness when the mind through calmness ceases to work—deeper than man-made awareness."

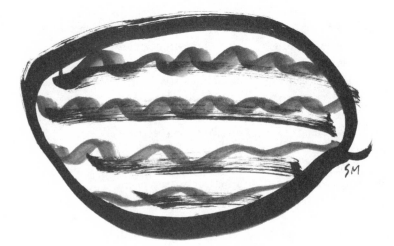

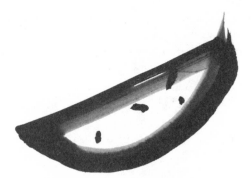

GRASP IT !
WITHOUT HANDS

Index

A

Acorn squash:
  in Coconut Curry Vegetables, 70
  in Roasted Autumn Vegetables, 128
  in Sweet Red Sauce, 162
  for tomatoes and zucchini *in* Tomato
    and Zucchini Primavera, 44
Aduki beans:
  Mixed Green Salad with, 141
  notes on, 211
  Spicy, 132
Agar-agar (kanten), notes on, 211
Almonds, *in* Linzertorte, 197
Apple(s):
  dried, *in* Hot Stewed Fruits with
    Ricotta, 184
  in Fruit Tart, 192
  in Hot Stewed Fruits with Ricotta,
    184
  for pears *in* Pear Custard Tart, 194
  Pie, Deep-Dish, 196
  for plums *in* Plum Torte, 198
  Pudding, 201
  Summer Mint and, Chutney, 72
Apricot(s):
  dried, *in* Hot Stewed Fruits with
    Ricotta, 184
  in Fruit Tart, 192
  in Hot Stewed Fruits with Ricotta,
    184
  Lime Chutney, 168
  for pears *in* Pear Custard Tart, 194
Arborio rice:
  notes on, 213
  in Risotto with Swiss Chard, 49
Arrowroot, notes on, 211
Arugula:
  in Carrot and Navy Bean Mixed
    Salad, 142

  in Mesclun Salad, 140
  in Mixed Greens with Zucchini,
    Red Pepper, and Sunflower
    Seeds, 142
Asian-Style Peanut Sauce, 165
Asparagus Risotto, 50
Avocado:
  in California-Style Sushi, 99
  in Cheese Enchiladas, 81
  in Guacamole, 87
  Jicama and, Salad, 143
  and Red Peppers, 154
  Tomato Salsa, and Black Olives,
    Tostadas with, 85
  in White Gazpacho, 28

B

Baked New Potatoes with Rosemary,
  121
Baked Tomatoes, 121
Balsamic vinegar, notes on, 211
Basic Olive Oil Dressing, 166
Basic Tomato Sauce, 161
Basil:
  Chili Lime, Dressing, 167
  Japanese Eggplants and, Rigatoni
    with, 41
  in Pesto, 164
  Sauce, Summer Vegetable Soup
    with, 21
  and Tomatoes, Polenta with, 55
  Tomatoes and, Bruschetta with,
    113
Basmati rice:
  in Asparagus Risotto, 50
  notes on, 213
Bean(s):
  aduki:
    notes on, 211

Swiss chard:
  Risotto with, 49
  and Tomato Tart, 116
Szechuan Green Beans and Soba, 39

T
Tacos, notes on, 214
Tahini:
  notes on, 214
  in Spicy Sesame Butter, 169
Tamari:
  in dipping sauce for sushi, 95
  notes on, 214
Tart(s):
  Fruit, 192
  Lemon, with Berries, 193
  Pastry:
    Sweet, 191
    Whole Wheat, 114
  Pear Custard, 194
  Pepper, 115
  Swiss Chard and Tomato, 116
Tasting, importance of, 5
Thai Carrot Salad with Peanuts,
    144
Thai Noodle Salad, 150
Tofu:
  and Chili Lime Basil Dressing,
    Broccoli Salad with, 143
  in Curry Vegetable Stew, 69
  Kale and, Pizza with, 110
  in Lentil Salad, 147
  in Mushroom Enchiladas with Red
    Pepper Sauce, 82
  in Mushroom Stroganoff, 45
  notes on, 214
  in Pepper Tart, 115
  to prepare, 8
  Salad, 145
  Scrambled, 182
  in Spinach Broccoli Lasagne, 43
  Stir-Fry, 133

  in Swiss Chard and Tomato Tart,
    116
  in Vietnamese Spring Rolls, 101–2
Tomatillos:
  notes on, 214
  in Salsa Verde, 83
Tomato(es):
  Baked, 121
  and Basil, Bruschetta with, 113
  Basil and, Polenta with, 55
  Broccoli, Shiitake, and, Salad, 152
  Broiled, with Cilantro Pesto, 121
  in Cheese Enchiladas, 81
  cherry, *in* Hot and Spicy Cajun
    Shish Kebabs, 127
  Coconut Raita, 74
  Marinated, 148
  Mushroom, Pizza, 107
  and Navy Bean Soup, 23
  in Potato Provençal, 125
  in Ratatouille, 131
  Salsa, 84
    Avocado, and Black Olives, Tosta-
      das with, 85
  Sauce:
    Basic, 161
    Spaghetti with, 38
  in Spicy Squash Stew, 71
  in Summer Garden Pizza, 108
  in Sweet Red Sauce, 162
  Swiss Chard and, Tart, 116
  and Zucchini Primavera, 44
Torte, Plum, 198
Tortillas:
  corn:
    in Bean Enchiladas, 81
    in Mushroom Enchiladas with Red
      Pepper Sauce, 82
    notes on, 214
    Steamed, 79
    wheat, *in* Refried Bean Burrito
      with Salsa Verde, 80

whole wheat:
  in Bean Enchiladas, 81
  in Huevos Rancheros, 183
  in Mushroom Enchiladas with Red
    Pepper Sauce, 82
  in Nachos, 89
  in Quesadillas, 86
  see also Tostadas
Tostadas, 85
  with Red Pepper Sauce, 85
  with Tomato Salsa, Avocado, and
    Black Olives, 85
Turnips, *in* Chili Stew, 79

U

Udon noodles:
  in Dashi, 27
  notes on, 212–13
  in Pasta with Cashew Ginger Sauce,
    38
  with Pesto, 38
Unsaturated oils, notes on, 213

V

Vegetable(s):
  Autumn, Roasted, 128
  Coconut, Curry, 70
  Curry, Stew, 69
  to prepare, 8
  to steam, 8–9
  Steamed, and Garlic Sauce, Pasta
    with, 40
  Stir-Fry Rice and, 51
  Summer, Soup, with Basil Sauce, 21
  see also names of specific vegetables
Vichyssoise, Sweet Potato, 29
Vietnamese Spring Rolls, 101–2
  to fry, 102
Vinaigrette, Orange Raspberry, 167
Vinegar(s):
  balsamic, notes on, 211
  rice, notes on, 213

W

Walnuts:
  Caramelized, 151
  in Linzertorte, 197
Wasabi:
  in dipping sauce for sushi, 95
  notes on, 214
  to prepare for sushi, 95
Watercress, *in* Fettuccine with Fresh
    Greens, 47
Wheat tortillas, *in* Refried Bean Bur-
    rito with Salsa Verde, 80
White Gazpacho, 28
Whole Wheat Pizza Dough, 106
Whole Wheat Tart Pastry, 114
Whole wheat tortillas:
  in Bean Enchiladas, 81
  in Mushroom Enchiladas with Red
    Pepper Sauce, 82
  in Nachos, 89
  in Quesadillas, 86
Wild Rice Pilaf, 59

Y

Yellow peppers. *See* Pepper(s)
Yellow summer squash:
  in Hot and Spicy Cajun Shish
    Kebabs, 127
  in Pesto Pizza, 109
  in Primavera Rice, 53
  in Tofu Salad, 145
Yogurt:
  -Orange Sauce, 179
  Raita:
    with Cucumber, 73
    with Ginger and Honey, 73
  in Tomato Coconut Raita, 74

Z

Zucchini:
  Fritters, 124
  in Hot and Spicy Cajun Shish
    Kebabs, 127

Let's Keep in Touch

I hope you enjoyed reading this book as much as I did writing it.

I'd love to hear from you. If you have any questions or comments, please feel free to write or call me. I'd especially appreciate hearing what parts of the book you enjoyed the most.

I enjoy speaking to groups, and I offer regular classes in cooking and sensory awareness in various locations around the country.

I also send out a regular letter to my friends and students. It's informal, filled with new recipes, the latest information on food and health, and short essays on living and sensing much like the ones in this book. If you call or send a self-addressed stamped envelope, I'll send you a copy of my latest letter.

It's been a pleasure spending this time with you. Let's keep in touch.

Sincerely,

Bettina Vitell
P. O. Box 273
2443 Fillmore Street
San Francisco, CA 94115
(415) 905-9524 (call anytime)